Practical Manual of
INTRAOCULAR
INFLAMMATION

Practical Manual of
INTRAOCULAR INFLAMMATION

Andrew D. Dick
University of Bristol
Bristol, UK

Annabelle A. Okada
Kyorin University School of Medicine
Tokyo, Japan

John V. Forrester
University of Aberdeen
Aberdeen, UK

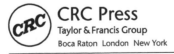

CRC Press
Taylor & Francis Group
Boca Raton London New York

CRC Press is an imprint of the
Taylor & Francis Group, an **informa** business

CRC Press
Taylor & Francis Group
6000 Broken Sound Parkway NW, Suite 300
Boca Raton, FL 33487-2742

First issued in paperback 2019

ISBN-13: 978-0-8493-9183-5 (hbk)
ISBN-13: 978-0-367-38720-4 (pbk)

Library of Congress Cataloging-in-Publication Data

Dick, Andrew.
    Practical manual of intraocular inflammation/Andrew D. Dick, Annabelle A. Okada, John V. Forrester.
       p. ; cm.
    Includes bibliographical references and index.
    ISBN-13: 978-0-8493-9183-5 (hardcover : alk. paper)
    ISBN-10: 0-8493-9183-0 (hardcover : alk. paper)
    1. Eye—Inflammation.   2. Uveitis. I. Forrester, John V. II. Okada, Annabelle. III. Title.
    [DNLM: 1. Uveitis—diagnosis.   2. Uveitis—therapy.   3. Inflammation—therapy. 4. Vision Disorders—prevention & control. WW 240 D547p 2008]
    RE96.D55 2008
    617.7′5—dc22

                                          2008008244

Visit the Taylor & Francis Web site at
http://www.taylorandfrancis.com

and the CRC Press Web site at
http://www.crcpress.com

Preface

There are many excellent examples of reference textbooks covering the bewildering clinical spectrum and complexity of the diagnosis and management of uveitis disorders. When faced with the uveitis patient in clinic, however, patients rarely present as per textbook diagnosis. So the challenge of uveitis requires a systematic approach to clinical assessment and interpretation of investigations to arrive at a management pathway suitable for that patient. This requires an ability to distinguish between infectious and noninfectious causes and the skill to recognize *sight-threatening* posterior segment inflammation. Alongside, there is a need to diagnose specific uveitic conditions and their association, or otherwise, with systemic disease for appropriate treatment in the longer term and being able to gauge an overall prognosis.

The purpose of this book is, therefore, by no means to compete with the excellent reference texts currently available, or the *update* texts that are frequently published and that hone in on specific *cutting-edge* overviews of specific aspects of uveitis. We rather wished to convey a book to complement such works. We feel there is a need to deliver a *handbook* that can provide a simplified synopsis of the more sight-threatening uveitis conditions, better termed posterior segment intraocular inflammatory disease. A book to fit in the pocket, keep handy in the briefcase, or sit on the office desk and help in the daily task of treating uveitis patients. As such, the book aims to deliver a background to and context of the clinical problems we face in managing patients with uveitis and systematically cover a practical approach to the management of the patient in clinic, while introducing treatment algorithms. We also show where we believe part of the future lies as a result of our increased understanding of the pathogenic mechanisms of disease alongside the explosion of specific immune therapies being developed for clinical use.

Given the increase in the pharmacopocias available and the increasingly robust evidence of their clinical efficacy, the delivery of "optimal" care remains challenging. To address some of the difficulties, we hope the book will assist training courses and modules/fellowships in ocular inflammation/uveitis available worldwide. In addition, dedicated accredited specialist training in medical ophthalmology, such as provided by the Royal College of Physicians in the United Kingdom, includes core training in uveitis and is breeding a new cadre of ophthalmic physicians specially trained in the diagnosis and management of ocular inflammatory diseases. We hope that the book will highlight an optimal approach as encouraged by specific training to generate recognized competence in both the diagnosis and monitoring of disease. This avoids the less definitive practice in which the institution and monitoring of the medical therapy is devolved to the internist or rheumatologist who may be less well placed to recognize improvement or worsening in the ocular condition, and so overall there is an arguable tendency never to achieve adequate control of ocular inflammation.

We dedicate the book to the memory of Professor Tetsuo Hida (1948–2008), Chairman of the Department of Ophthalmology, Kyorin University School of Medicine. Professor Hida was a world-renown vitreoretinal surgeon and past-president of the Japanese Ophthalmological Society. He will be remembered by a generation of young Japanese ophthalmologists who were fortunate enough to be graced by his knowledge, wisdom, and generosity.

Andrew D. Dick
Annabelle A. Okada
John V. Forrester

Acknowledgments

We are indebted to the help and support of all our colleagues in our respective uveitis services, for their cumulative thoughts over the years, which when distilled have contributed greatly to the genesis of this book. This ongoing dialogue, we hope, has been represented in this practical management handbook. We would also like to thank our fellows in uveitis for their hard work and support and in particular Drs. Lucia Kuffova and Susan Kelly for preparing many of the figures alongside our respective staff from ophthalmic photography departments for their excellence, particularly Ms. Sumie Minemura, Ms. Nozomi Watanabe, Mr. Steve Nielson, and Mrs. Alison Farrow. Also thanks to Dr. Lindsay Nicholson, who generated some of the figures representing immune responses in chapter 1.

Contents

1

What Are We Dealing With?

Uveitis, although comparatively rare when compared with diabetic retinopathy, for example, remains a significant cause of visual handicap in the working age population (1). The reasons often relate to the difficulty in the clinic in ascertaining sight-threatening disease, treating aggressively enough to prevent irreversible retinal damage or chronic blood-ocular barrier breakdown and macular edema.

UVEITIS—POSTERIOR SEGMENT
INTRAOCULAR INFLAMMATION (PSII)

Uveitis is an encompassing term for inflammation within the eye, which includes many disease entities, either infectious or (auto)immune mediated. Although the various forms of uveitis are anatomically described, we often use terms interchangeably and inconsistently, such as *iritis, anterior uveitis, iridocyclitis, vitritis, intermediate uveitis, posterior uveitis, chorioretinitis*, and *panuveitis*. Immediately, one gets a feeling of difference of opinion and lack of understanding simply because of lack of clarity of definitions used. Besides, many uveitic entities are associated with systemic immune-mediated disorders, most commonly, B27-related spondyloarthropathies, sarcoidosis, multiple sclerosis, and Behçet's disease. Given such heterogeneity of disorders within an overarching term such as *uveitis*, the International Ocular Inflammation Society has coined the term *posterior segment intraocular inflammation* (PSII), which better describes the embracing phenotype of the more sight-threatening conditions we encounter in clinic.

1

Table 1 The SUN Working Group Anatomic Classification of Uveitis

Type	Primary site of inflammation[a]	Includes
Anterior uveitis	Anterior chamber	Iritis Iridocyclitis Anterior cyclitis
Intermediate uveitis	Vitreous	Pars planitis Posterior cyclitis Hyalitis
Posterior uveitis	Retina or choroid	Focal, multifocal, or diffuse choroiditis Chorioretinitis Retinochoroiditis Retinitis Neuroretinitis
Panuveitis	Anterior chamber, vitreous, and retina or choroid	

[a]As determined clinically.
Abbreviation: SUN, standardization of uveitis nomenclature.
Source: Adapted from Bloch-Michel E, Nussenblatt RB. International Uveitis Study Group recommendations for the evaluation of intraocular inflammatory disease. Am J Ophthalmol 1987; 103:234–235.

Standardization of Uveitis Nomenclature

When an international working group met and was surveyed about diagnostic terminology and grading of inflammation, the outcome, reported in *American Journal of Ophthalmology* (2), proposed terminologies to standardize our description of uveitis (Table 1). While this classification remains anatomical, a reductionist approach allows other uveitic synonyms to be incorporated within each and reduce potential confusion. This approach is without compromise to the diagnostic ability of underlying systemic immune-mediated disorders or to overall patient treatment. The classification also recognizes the frequent overlap on presentation of the phenotype PSII by amalgamating previous terms for uveitis into simplified anatomical groups. This helps concentrate one of the main decision processes on the initial patient assessment as to where anatomically the primary site of inflammation lies, how likely infectious etiology is, and how sight-threatening the inflammation is (Figs. 1 and 2).

Further recommendations of this working party were given regarding standardization, in particular, the extent of inflammation and definition of relapse or remission. Such definitions are not only very useful toward standardizing the reporting of clinical studies but also for everyday clinical practice and will be highlighted later when we expand on our practical management guide for the management of PSII.

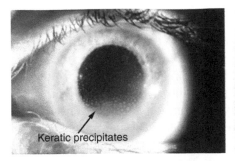
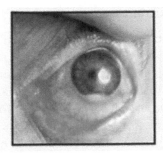

Figure 1 Clinical photographs of acute anterior uveitis. These clinical pictures demonstrate keratic precipitates (*left*) and in more severe cases, hypopyon (*right*). These signs can be observed in any form of anterior uveitis (e.g., HLA-B27-related, Behçet's disease, herpetic) or as a feature of more significant sight-threatening disease in intermediate uveitis, posterior uveitis, or panuveitis.

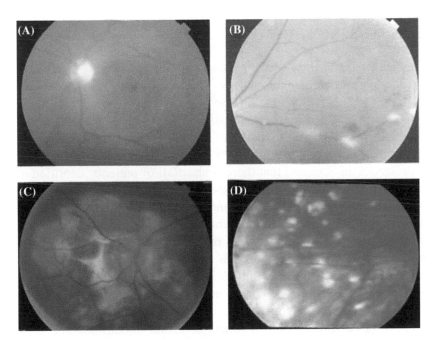

Figure 2 Clinical Color fundal photographs of various forms of PSII. (**A**): Vitreous haze in presence of predominant feature of vitritis in patient with intermediate uveitis. (B–D): Features of posterior uveitis. (**B**): Perivascular cuffing in patient with retinal vasculitis secondary to sarcoidosis. (**C**): Chorioretinitis and peripapillary subretinal fibrosis due to peripapillary choroidal neovascularization secondary to serpiginous choroidopathy. (**D**): Multifocal chorioretinal lesions in patient with idiopathic multifocal chorioretinitis.

Disease Burden

Although incidence and prevalence of disease varies throughout the world, as does the underlying etiology, with respect to infection, there is increasing awareness of the socioeconomic burden of PSII (3). There are many studies to show the differences in types of uveitis and their causes. Comparison worldwide is difficult because of the lack of uniformity of terminology used. What can be said is that the prevalence of uveitis is increasing. Globally, the prevalence and incidence figures are hard to gauge as many reports are not population based and toward tertiary referral centers. Because, until recently, there was a lack of consensus definitions (2), most studies are not centered on well-defined diagnostic criteria or classification of uveitis. However, despite that, recent comparative patterns of the epidemiology of uveitis (4) have shown a changing pattern of uveitic etiology within regions over time. Not surprisingly, however, in tropical countries, there remains a high prevalence of infectious uveitis.

WHAT ARE WE DEALING WITH?

It is well recognized that the majority of cases of uveitis presenting to tertiary referral clinics do not reflect the burden or frequency of uveitis entities in community practice (5). Nevertheless, in the United States, for example, a population-based study revealed a prevalence of 115.3/100,000 and incidence of 52.4/100,000 patients (6), providing evidence of a much greater burden of disease than previous estimates. Compounding this is the suggestion from data from National Health Service in Scotland that there is shortfall of patients identified at risk and receiving appropriate immunosuppressive therapy (7). The impact of uveitis in blindness of course varies globally and will be region-dependent. What remains for both developed and developing countries is the significant adverse socioeconomic impact of loss of vision. It remains likely that the estimate, although now old figures, of a baseline 6% of middle-aged people visually impaired due to uveitis in developed countries is an underestimate. What is still recognized is that chronic PSII-related cystoid macular edema is a major cause of visual loss. Although studies are retrospective in hospital tertiary referral–based surveys, up to 35% of patients exhibit blindness or visual impairment and 23% require one or more surgical interventions (1,8). The impact of uveitis remains unknown yet is likely to stay significant, accounting for approximately 5% to 20% of cases of legal blindness in developed countries.

Studies show that the majority (over 90%) of uveitis cases in the community remain anterior uveitis, whereas in tertiary practice there is a high prevalence of sight-threatening PSII (up to 50%). In developed countries, infectious causes of or systemic disorders associated with uveitis account for approximately 50% of cases, the commonest of which are human leukocyte antigen (HLA)-B27-associated anterior uveitis and toxoplasma chorioretinitis, a remarkably equal split between immune-mediated noninfectious and infectious etiology!

REGIONAL DIFFERENCES

Infections

As one can imagine, there are marked differences in infectious causes of uveitis globally. Infectious uveitis in the developed world is for the most part secondary to *toxoplasmosis* with other causes being caused by herpesviruses. Less common infections include tuberculosis, syphilis, Lyme disease, and Bartonellosis. Of course, even infectious causes in developed countries vary regionally, depending on the prevalence of individual infectious agents, such as *Borrelia burgdorferi* or *histoplasma* within different areas of United States or, for example, high prevalence of toxoplasmosis in South America. Similar trends are seen in developing countries with higher incidences such as onchocerciasis in West Africa. In India, reports comment particularly on a remarkably high incidence of tuberculosis but also syphilis and leprosy. In more recent reports, up to 30% of uveitis cases were secondary to infection. What is common to all studies, when comparing countries and moreover districts within large countries, are the pronounced regional differences in infectious causes with respect to (*i*) age and demographics of population—infections in developing countries, particularly parasitic, have been reported to be more common in children, (*ii*) whether the infectious agent is endemic in a region (e.g., *Toxoplasma*, Borrelia, HTLV-1, and *Onchocerca*), and (*iii*) the prevalence of HIV/AIDS. Another compounding factor is the prevalence of HIV and AIDS within the region and community, which will skew the infectious causes of uveitis. So in the absence of a successful antiretroviral program, there are higher incidences, for example, of CMV (cytomegalovirus) retinitis and *toxoplasma* chorioretinitis.

Noninfectious Uveitis

Again, considerable variation between countries exists. In most studies, seronegative spondyloarthropathy–associated uveitis is the most common, except for example, in Japan, although the prevalence is increasing. When considering causes of uveitis, there are distinct demographic differences. For example, studies show that sarcoidosis remains relatively uncommon in Italy, Israel, and China compared with northern Europe or United States, whereas Behçet's disease is a leading cause of sight-threatening PSII in Turkey, China, Saudi Arabia, and Israel, and comparatively rare in Northern Europe. The differences may be accounted for by underlying genetic predisposition (see below), as we recognize that specific HLA allelic associations with Vogt-Koyanagi-Harada syndrome (VKH) and Behçet's disease are more prevalent within individual populations.

Given the differences between regions, it is important to recognize the epidemiological data for each region and to have knowledge practicing in different regions of the predominant forms of uveitis in each area when considering a differential diagnosis.

HOW SHOULD WE CLASSIFY OUR PATIENTS?

The conflict between anatomical classification, presence or absence of systemic disease, presence or absence of infection, and giving the disease a name is important to define and resolve. However, we will be informing a practical management that will in part use established classification systems that assist in defining disease and potentially identifying patients at risk of *sight-threatening* disease or a more chronic protracted disease course, leading to visual loss. The SUN guidelines described above (2) deliver in part this recognition of at least generating a classification of uveitis and how to report case cohorts. In practice, however, we still do not have a composite scoring system (analogous to rheumatological disorders) that permits accurate representation of severity of disease or correlates with short- or long-term prognosis. On the other hand, the diagnosis of certain uveitic entities is assisted by published international criteria, and we will be referring to these. For example, in Behçet's disease, the *international criteria* include recurrent oral ulceration, plus two of the following:

- Recurrent genital ulcerations
- Eye lesions (anterior uveitis or posterior uveitis)
- Cells in the vitreous
- Retinal vasculitis
- Skin lesions (erythema nodosum, pseudofolliculitis, papulopustular lesions, acneiform nodules in a postadolescent patient not taking corticosteroids)
- Positive pathergy test

For VKH, a recently revised international criterion has been published (chap. 3, Table 3) (9), defining complete and incomplete syndromes. This criterion is useful for diagnostic purposes, however, in practice it has been questioned as to the sensitivity of making the diagnosis early in disease presentation. So while striving to make a diagnosis, the efforts should not

Table 2 Classifications of Childhood Arthritis

ACR (1977)	EULAR (1978)	ILAR (1997)
Juvenile rheumatoid arthritis (JRA)	Juvenile chronic arthritis (JCA)	Juvenile idiopathic arthritis (JIA)
Systemic	Systemic	Systemic
Polyarticular	Polyarticular Juvenile rheumatoid arthritis	Polyarticular RF-negative Polyarticular RF-positive
Pauciarticular	Pauciarticular	Oligoarticular Persistent Extended
	Juvenile psoriatic arthritis Juvenile ankylosing spondylitis	Psoriatic arthritis Enthesitis-related arthritis Other arthritis

Abbreviations: ACR, American College of Rheumatology; EULAR, European League Against Rheumatism; ILAR, International League of Associations for Rheumatology; RF, rheumatoid factor.

preclude accurate assessment as to severity of inflammation and more importantly, instituting appropriate immunosuppressive therapy.

The same can be said when considering a more pragmatic practical management of uveitis associated with juvenile idiopathic arthritis (JIA) and combining the classification of JIA for research purposes (10). Despite numerous classifications, prognostically, for uveitis the data only support that the children most at risk remain those who present with early-onset aggressive disease and pauciarticular arthritis (Table 2). The prognostic value of antinuclear antibody (ANA) and female sex remains unconfirmed with different cohorts reporting ANA of no prognostic value and a worse disease occurring in males in other studies.

IMMUNOPATHOLOGY OF NONINFECTIOUS PSII

What Triggers Uveitis?

In the absence of overt infectious causes, PSII occurs as a result of autoinflammatory (autoimmune) responses against our own tissues. As highlighted above, broadly 50% of noninfectious autoinflammatory PSII are limited to the eye and the remainder form part of more generalized systemic disorders. However, there is noticeable overlap. While it is clear that infectious agents must be excluded before commencing immunosuppressive therapy (e.g., *toxoplasmosis,* herpetic retinopathies, syphilis, etc.), as we will detail later in the book, the distinction can be difficult as infectious disease can mimic autoinflammatory disease (e.g., Lyme disease and intermediate uveitis). Also, immunologically,

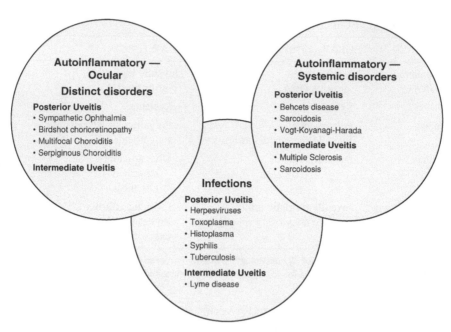

Figure 3 Overlap between autoinflammatory ocular and autoinflammatory systemic disease and infection.

immune responses to infectious or noninfectious causes are not too dissimilar, and indeed, infections may be central to the initiation and/or perpetuation of autoinflammatory disorders (Fig. 3).

The clinical features of PSII tell us little of the underlying immunopathology of these conditions, and consensus deriving data from experimental models and the clinic is that in the majority, noninfectious PSII forms part of a spectrum of autoimmune responses possessing common immune and tissue-damaging effector mechanisms. It is armed with such increased understanding of immune mechanisms that we are developing improved management pathways and treatments, which we will cover throughout the book for these blinding conditions, and look into the future with new approaches toward developing therapies.

Immunity and the Autoinflammatory Response

Immunity has developed to combat the harmful effects of infection and the taking over of our genome with the introduction of foreign genes. To achieve this requires an ability to kill and then responses fine-tuned with memory to rapidly attack repeated invasions. To achieve such a capacity, the immune system has cross talk between the *innate* and *acquired* (memory) immune responses. We have developed innate barriers, such as skin, blood barriers, and those pertinent to the eye—lids, tears, mucin, and an arguably sequestered and protected intraocular environment resulting from defined blood-ocular barriers and lack of anatomically defined lymphatic drainage. Moreover, there are a plethora of cells that can report injury/inflammation (epithelial cells, mast cells, macrophages, neutrophils, platelets, and endothelial cells). ***So what triggers an immune response?*** There have been several theories that have evolved: the *danger* theory purports that injured host cells release alarm signals that activate antigen-presenting cells (APC) [and for the eye, this includes dendritic cells (DC) in the choroid and macrophages in iris and retina]; the *pattern recognition* theory infers that microbial "non-self" antigens induce an innate response, which, in turn, triggers an acquired response; and finally, *ongoing binary signaling*, which is a view where a normal immune response results from the ongoing detection of either signal that reports injury or signals that report infection. In all theories, T cells are central to the adaptive immune response. Their activation depends on signals through the T-cell receptor (TCR) and their responses are modified by a range of co-stimulatory signals. *So how do we bridge the first line of defense against invading pathogens and trigger the acquired immune response?* Toll-like receptor (TLR) family is expressed on our immune cells and recognizes conserved motifs on invading pathogens. TLR ligation on professional APC, such as DC, facilitates their maturation, activation, and migration from tissue to regional lymph nodes, where T-cell activation occurs. Hence, TLR (innate activation) has the ability to bridge innate and acquired immune responses by mobilizing adaptive immunity, and principally, Th1 responses (see below). Further forms of pathogen-associated molecular pattern (PAMPs) recognition, other than TLR ligation, include the intracytoplasmic nod-like receptors. Mutations in NOD2 genes (CARD15), for example, give rise to an autoinflammatory state known as Blau's syndrome (patients may have uveitis), and which may mimic infantile sarcoidosis and gives rise to cellular infiltration including T cells in tissues. Mutations in CARD15 gene occur in patients with Crohn's disease, an inflammatory bowel disease where patients may generate uveitis.

As a result of APC activation and interaction with $CD4^+$ T cells, T cells polarize into three main classes: Th1, Th17, and Th2 (Fig. 4), which are defined by their canonical signature cytokines they release, and polarization is dependent on the peptide and cytokine signals they receive when interacting with the APC.

In the context of PSII and autoinflammatory disease, $CD4^+$ T cells, which recognize self-antigens, are either normally deleted by clonal selection in the thymus during development or, escaping this, are subsequently controlled by tolerance/regulatory mechanisms in the periphery. It is a breakdown of such regulation that putatively generates pathogenic autoinflammatory responses. Regulation of possible autoinflammatory T-cell responses is afforded by the

T cell activation

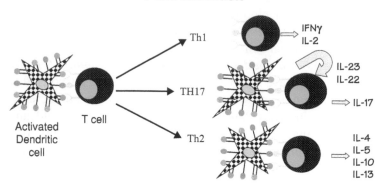

Figure 4 Activation and polarization of T-cell responses. T cells are activated by receptor-ligand interactions in what is known as the immunological synapse. Antigen is processed by the DC, peptides of which are presented to T cells within the MHC groove on the DC, which is recognized by TCR. For CD4$^+$ T-cell activation, this involves MHC class II molecules. For full T-cell activation, peptide presentation occurs alongside co-stimulation via other receptor-ligand interactions, such as CD28-B7 and CD40L-CD40. Once T-cell activation occurs, their polarization and function are identified by cytokines they release. *Abbreviations*: DC, dendritic cells; MHC, major histocompatability complex; TCR, T-cell receptor.

presence of naturally occurring regulatory T cells (Treg cells). Over time, there have been many regulatory phenotypes described, some of which are naturally occurring and others that are induced following antigen recognition (Fig. 5) (11).

Irrespective of which triggering event breaks the regulation, antigen-specific CD4$^+$ T cells can initiate disease only after peripheral clonal expansion and probably on further presentation of antigen either in regional drainage lymph nodes or at the target tissue (Fig. 6).

Initiation of autoinflammation is subclinical. Once symptomatic, it is likely that the majority of the responses we see clinically in the eye are nonspecific inflammation and chronic (Fig. 7). There may be additional local cellular and molecular immune regulatory mechanisms also acting to reduce the bystander collateral damage on the background of a reduced but constant antigen-specific response.

Evidence for Autoinflammatory Disease

As we have discussed above, the general view is that PSII is regarded as a CD4$^+$ T cell–mediated disease where activated T cells can be detected in the peripheral blood as well as ocular fluids of patients with uveitis. There is no definitive evidence for autoimmunity, hence, the more accepted term *autoinflammatory*, where the evidence is compelling in comparison with only circumstantial evidence of true autoimmunity (Table 3). Studies show that in the peripheral blood, there are markers of immune activation, including vascular endothelial

Regulatory cells

■ Naturally occurring or induced T cell populations

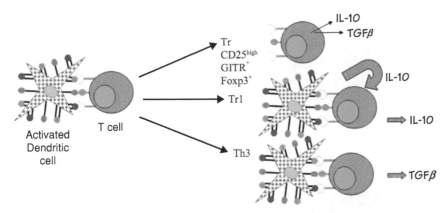

Figure 5 Classes of regulatory T cells. Natural Tr cells develop in the thymus, their TCR repertoire is mainly self-reactive, and the expression of Foxp3$^+$ determines their regulatory function. In human disease IPEX, there are mutations in Foxp3. There is, however, diversity in regulatory cells. Tr1 cells (Foxp3^{neg}) and Th3 cells, which are induced following antigen exposure and regulate as a result of their signature cytokines they generate (IL-10 and TGFβ, respectively). *Abbreviations*: TCR, T-cell receptor; IPEX, immune dysfunction/polyendocrinopathy/enteropathy/x-linked.

Table 3 Evidence of Immune Activation in Patients with Noninfectious Uveitis

Autoimmunity and T-cell activation in uveitis

- Peripheral T-cell activation (IL-2r, CD69)
- Immune activation upregulation of adhesion molecules and selectins
- Association with HLA-DR15, HLA-DR4
- Tyrosinase-specific CD4$^+$ T cell in VKH
- S-Ag-specific T cell in uveitis
- Clinical response to anti-T-cell agents (e.g., CsA and anti-TAC)

activation, the presence of autoreactive tyrosinase-related protein–specific T cells in VKH as well as S-Ag-specific T-cell responses and S-Ag-specific autoantibodies, particularly, for example, in Birdshot chorioretinopathy. More recently, there is data that supports increased Th17 responses in the peripheral blood of VKH patients as well as other forms of uveitis and scleritis, which, like the interferon-gamma Th1 T-cell counterpart, is IL-2-dependent as the cells' growth factor (12). We also know that there is a significant association of PSII phenotypes with HLA-major histocompatability complex (HLA-MHC) class II

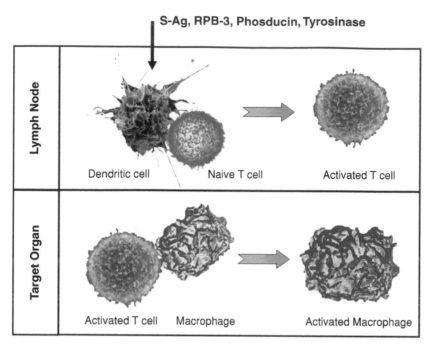

S-Ag, RPB-3, Phosducin, Tyrosinase

Figure 6 Activation of an autoinflammatory response. Activated DC traffic to the regional lymph nodes where the DC will present peptides of putative ocular autoantigens (S-antigen, retinoid-binding protein, phosducin, or tyrosinase-related proteins) to T cells, generating activated antigen-specific CD4$^+$ T cells. Antigen-specific CD4$^+$ T cells home back to the eye where further interaction with resident and infiltrating myeloid cells activates macrophages that contribute to the autoinflammatory tissue damage. *Abbreviation*: DC, dendritic cells.

alleles, implicating CD4$^+$ T-cell activation in the pathogenesis of disease (Table 4) (13). This is particularly so for PSII related with systemic disease, such as VKH, JIA-associated uveitis, tubulointerstitial nephritis and uveitis (TINU), and intermediate uveitis. The association with HLA-DR antigens are similar to that described for other autoinflammatory conditions such as rheumatoid arthritis, inflammatory bowel disease, diabetes mellitus, and multiple sclerosis. The significance of the HLA association between different populations depends on the prevalence of the relevant gene in the population. This is true even for different HLA-DR associations being reported for different populations (e.g., sympathetic ophthalmia with DRB1*0405 in Asians and *0404 in Europeans). Extending the role of genetic influences in autoinflammatory disease, there has been increasing interest in the understanding of Class III MHC genes, or cytokine and chemokine polymorphisms in generating evidence for predicting predisposition, severity, and course of disease. These include polymorphisms in tumor necrosis factor (TNF) and TNF receptor genes, IL-10, interferon-gamma, and chemokines such as

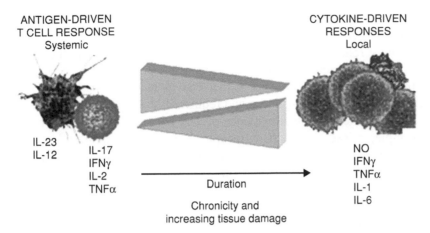

Figure 7 Engaging a non-antigen-specific response contributing to tissue damage. Following initial activation of APC (DC) and then trafficking to lymph node, the early event of antigen-specific T-cell activation and proliferation is with time diluted by the pro-inflammatory cascade. With increasing chronicity of disease, more nonspecific T-cell activation and macrophage activation within the target tissue occurs. Activation of macrophages and other myeloid cells (mast cells, neutrophils) gives rise to the tissue damage we observe clinically, mediated by reactive oxygen species, nitric oxide, and direct cytolytic effect of some of the cytokines generated by both the myeloid and T cells. *Abbreviations*: APC, antigen-presenting cells; DC, dendritic cells.

Table 4 HLA Associations with Noninfectious Ocular Inflammatory Conditions

Disease	HLA
Acute Anterior Uveitis	B27
Behçet's Disease	B51
Birdshot Chorioretinopathy	A29
Intermediate Uveitis	DR15
Juvenile Idiopathic Arthritis	DPB1*0102
Sympathetic Ophthalmia	DRB*0104, DRB*0105, DQA1*03
TINU	DRB1*0102
VKH syndrome	DR1, DR4 (DRB1*0405)

Abbreviations: TINU, tubulointerstitial nephritis and uveitis; VKH, Vogt-Koyanagi-Harada syndrome; HLA, human leukocyte antigen.

CXCR1, CXCR2, CCL2, and CCL5 in studies of various cohorts of patients including Behçet's disease, sympathetic ophthalmia, intermediate uveitis, and retinal vasculitis. Although in general, the data is not robust to accurately predict, there is ever increasing evidence supporting the influence genetic polymorphisms have in the severity and course of uveitis. For example, specific mutations can lead to hypersecretion of cytokines such as mutations in cold autoinflammatory syndrome 1 (CIAS1) gene that encodes cryopyrin and leads to hypersecretion of IL-1 and conditions related to ocular inflammation such as chronic infantile neurological, cutaneous, articular (CINCA) syndrome.

Archetypically, one current concept is that PSII is mediated by Th1 CD4$^+$ T cells, which generate interferon-gamma and require IL-2 as an essential growth factor. Consequently, one can detect evidence of Th1 activation in the peripheral blood, for example, raised serum IL-2 receptor levels, and increased CD69 expression on T cells. More recently, there is evidence for Th17 activation and upregulation of cell numbers in uveitis patients. What is manifest and supports a T cell–driven disease is the response to therapy of specific T-cell calcineurin inhibitors such as cyclosporin or tacrolimus and, most recently, specific IL-2 receptor blockade (anti-TAC).

PRACTICAL CLASSIFICATION FOR MANAGEMENT

Throughout the handbook, we will emphasize a practical view of classifying patients to assist their management and develop schema to follow to assist diagnosis and treatment of *sight-threatening* disease. The concept follows: examination of patients for both ocular and systemic manifestations of inflammatory disease (and other comorbid disease states), a decision (and this may require support from laboratory and imaging investigation) as to whether PSII is infective or noninfective, and finally, whether the patient has sight-threatening disease or not. This initial clinical assessment determines the appropriate treatment at the outset, which can be modified when further results arrive or changes occur clinically.

REFERENCES

1. Rothova A, Suttorp-van Schulten MS, Frits Treffers W, et al. Causes and frequency of blindness in patients with intraocular inflammatory disease. Br J Ophthalmol 1996; 80(4):332–336.

2. Jabs DA, Nussenblatt RB, Rosenbaum JT. Standardization of uveitis nomenclature for reporting clinical data. Results of the First International Workshop. Am J Ophthalmol 2005; 140(3):509–516.

3. Suttorp-Schulten MS, Rothova A. The possible impact of uveitis in blindness: a literature survey. Br J Ophthalmol 1996; 80(9):844–848.

4. Rathinam SR, Namperumalsamy P. Global variation and pattern changes in epidemiology of uveitis. Indian J Ophthalmol 2007; 55(3):173–183.

5. McCannel CA, Holland GN, Helm CJ, et al. Causes of uveitis in the general practice of ophthalmology. UCLA Community-Based Uveitis Study Group. Am J Ophthalmol 1996; 121(1):35–46.

6. Gritz DC, Wong IG. Incidence and prevalence of uveitis in Northern California; the Northern California Epidemiology of Uveitis Study. Ophthalmology 2004; 111(3): 491–500; discussion 500.

7. Williams GJ, Brannan S, Forrester JV, et al. The prevalence of sight-threatening uveitis in Scotland. Br J Ophthalmol 2007; 91(1):33–36.

8. Lardenoye CW, van Kooij B, Rothova A. Impact of macular edema on visual acuity in uveitis. Ophthalmology 2006; 113(8):1446–1449.

9. Rao NA, Sukavatcharin S, Tsai JH. Vogt-Koyanagi-Harada disease diagnostic criteria. Int Ophthalmol 2007; 27(2–3):195–199.

10. Duffy CM, Colbert RA, Laxer RM, et al. Nomenclature and classification in chronic childhood arthritis: time for a change? Arthritis Rheum 2005; 52(2):382–385.

11. Rouse BT. Regulatory T cells in health and disease. J Intern Med 2007; 262(1): 78–95.

12. Amadi-Obi A, Yu CR, Liu X, et al. TH17 cells contribute to uveitis and scleritis and are expanded by IL-2 and inhibited by IL-27/STAT1. Nat Med 2007; 13(6):711–718.

13. Levinson RD. Immunogenetics of ocular inflammatory disease. Tissue Antigens 2007; 69(2):105–112.

What Are We Dealing With

2

Clinical Assessment of Patients with Posterior Segment Intraocular Inflammation

GENERAL FEATURES AND CLINICAL EVALUATION OF INTRAOCULAR INFLAMMATION IN THE CLINIC

The cardinal features of intraocular inflammation are cellular infiltrate and breakdown of the blood ocular barrier, and are characterized clinically as *vitritis*, *retinal vasculitis*, and *chorioretinitis*. Clinically, one issue that remains is to define active versus inactive disease. While this can be extremely straightforward for conditions such as *panuveitis* or *intermediate uveitis* (predominant vitritis), it can be more difficult because of clinical subtleties for chorioretinitis and retinal vasculitis. In this chapter, we will first describe the clinical features of active and inactive posterior segment intraocular inflammation (PSII) before going on to give overviews of signs that may lead us to describe infectious versus noninfectious disease and determine sight-threatening disease. Such features will be further emphasized in chapter 3, where we will hone down on describing diagnosis and management of specific infectious and noninfectious PSII, and how the clinical feature may assist in driving toward a specific diagnosis. To this end, in this chapter we will describe the general systemic overview examination of patients with uveitis, including supporting imaging and laboratory investigations.

CLINICAL EVALUATION—SYMPTOMS AND SIGNS

Defining Clinical Onset and Course of Uveitis—Standardized Nomenclature

Although the Standardised Uveitis Nomenclature (SUN) working group reported on consensus nomenclature for reporting studies of uveitis, in our mind, it forms good practice for the daily clinical management of patients. Therefore, descriptors of onset and course of uveitis are important in defining patients' clinical presentation and understanding where the patient is in the course of disease; irrespective of underlying etiology or pathogenesis. This is summarized in Table 1 (1).

Defining Active Disease

Anterior Segment Inflammation
Clinical signs and symptoms are important differentiators of anterior segment inflammation (Box 1), and although we are predominantly dealing with management of PSII in this book, it is necessary to determine the extent and grade of anterior segment inflammation (which may of course occur alone, and we will be highlighting that throughout the book) or PSII, especially, intermediate uveitis and panuveitis. Recent consensus has adapted previous scoring systems, but essentially, it remains that cardinal activity signs are those of *cells* in and *flare* of the aqueous [Table 2, as adapted from (1)].

Vitritis
Vitritis refers to inflammation in the vitreous gel and is assessed by the extent of cellular infiltration in the vitreous. Often in mild cases, this may be asymptomatic. Otherwise, patients will frequently complain of floaters, which, if significant, make the vision "blurred" or reduced on acuity measurement. In blurring of or reduced vision, there is a need to determine whether this is due to significant

Table 1 The SUN Working Group Descriptors of Uveitis

Category	Descriptor	Comment
Onset	Sudden	
	Insidious	
Duration	Limited	≤3 months duration
	Persistent	>3 months duration
Course	Acute	Episode characterized by sudden onset and limited duration
	Recurrent	Repeated episodes separated by periods of inactivity without treatment ≥3 months in duration
	Chronic	Persistent uveitis with relapse in <3 months after discontinuing treatment

Abbreviation: SUN, standardization of uveitis nomenclature.

Box 1 Uveitis: Differential Symptoms and Signs					
Pain	**Redness/Injection**	**Corneal Haze**	**Discharge**	**Vision**	**Diagnosis**
None→mild	Pericorneal, none	Minimal	No	Blurred	Uveitis
None→FB	Peripheral/diffuse	No	Yellow	Normal	Conjunctivitis (bacterial)
Sensation/itch	Peripheral/diffuse	No	Watery	Normal	Conjunctivitis (viral)
	Peripheral/diffuse	No	No	Normal	Conjunctivitis (allergic)
Severe/boring	Sectoral/diffuse	No	No	Normal	Scleritis
Severe/headache	Pericorneal	Yes	No	Lost	Acute glaucoma
Severe/eye closing	Pericorneal	Yes	No	Lost	Keratitis/corneal ulcer
Severe/periocular	None	No	No/yes	Normal	Orbital cellulitis

Table 2 The SUN Working Group Grading Scheme for Anterior Chamber Cells and Flare

Grade	Cells in field[a]
0	<1
0.5+	1–5
1+	6–15
2+	16–25
3+	26–50
4+	>50

Grade	Description
0	None
1+	Faint
2+	Moderate (iris and lens details clear)
3+	Marked (iris and lens details hazy)
4+	Intense (fibrin or plastic aqueous)

[a]Field size is a 1 mm × 1 mm slit beam.
Abbreviation: SUN, standardization of uveitis nomenclature.

vitritis and opacities or due to *sight-threatening* disease with, for example, central retinal vasculitis or cystoid macular edema. How to determine *sight-threatening disease [sight-threatening ocular inflammation (STOI)]* will be discussed later. Scoring of vitritis is potentially fraught with error. Although *any* presence of vitreous cells is important, the counting of cells is difficult and error-prone on repeated examinations, and the presence of cells within the formed vitreous gel may not represent *active* disease, particularly in the presence of a recent acute posterior vitreous detachment as a result of previous but now largely resolved inflammation. A good schema for clinical practice is the National Eye Institute system for grading vitreous haze (Table 3, Fig. 1). It is now generally perceived

Table 3 Grading of Vitreous Haze Through the Binocular Indirect Ophthalmoscope (BIO SCORE)

Score	Description	Clinical findings
0	Nil	None
0.5	Trace	Occasional cells
1	Minimal	Posterior pole clearly visible
2	Mild	Posterior pole details slightly hazy
3	Moderate	Posterior pole details very hazy
4	Marked	Posterior pole details barely visible
5	Severe	Fundal details not visible

Source: Adapted from Ref. 2.

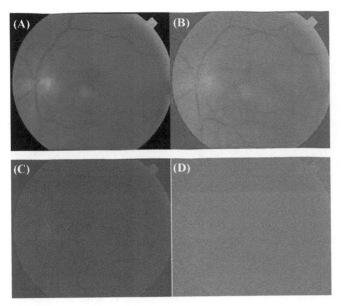

Figure 1 Binocular indirect ophthalmoscopic grading of vitreal haze (2). This composite fundus color image has been photographically enhanced to demonstrate the effects of vitritis/vitreal haze. (**A**) Normal view (grade 0). (**B**) Hazy view of posterior pole (grade 2). (**C**) Increasingly difficult to discern retinal vascular features (grade 3). (**D**) Barely visible retinal structures (grade 4).

that *pars planitis* should be used for that subset of intermediate uveitis (with predominant inflammation in the vitreous) where there is *snowbank* formation, in the absence of associated infection of systemic disease.

Symptoms   Vitritis, which is the predominant site of inflammation in intermediate uveitis, may be asymptomatic. However, when in context of panuveitis or retinal vasculitis, vitritis may also present with loss of vision (see below). In general, vitritis gives rise to the following symptoms:

- Floaters
- Blurring of vision, which may change with posture or eye movements and may effect stereopsis
- Reduced vision in case of significant vitreous opacity or in presence of acute posterior vitreous detachment

Clinical assessment   Of course, the clarity of visualizing the posterior pole with a 20-Dioptre or 90-Dioptre Lens via indirect biomicroscopy will depend on both the clarity of the cornea and the presence of cataract. Therefore, all binocular indirect ophthalmoscopy (BIO) score assessments (2) of vitreous haze should also be made in conjunction with cataract assessment [e.g., *lens opacity classification* (LOCS) III (3)].

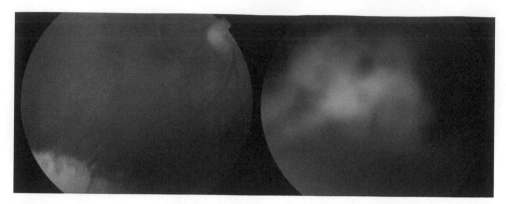

Figure 2 Fundus color photographs showing snowbanking in pars planitis. A snowbank in the inferotemporal peripheral retina (*right*). In extreme cases (*left*), snowbanking may extend and associated retinal vasculitis and leakage create exudation and subretinal fluid. The ensuing detachment may encroach to the macula and reduce vision.

Vitreous cells are best seen with *slit-lamp biomicroscopy*, with or without additional lens systems to view the posterior vitreous. On examination, you may note *anterior vitreous cells* (pertaining to those cells in retrolental space) and *posterior vitreous cells* in the cortical gel and in presence of posterior vitreous detachment in the retrohyaloid space. A classical sign, for example, of intermediate uveitis is *snowballs*, where large cellular aggregates accumulate inferiorly in the posterior vitreous gel. In extreme cases, there is a cellular and glial accumulation on the pars plana and anterior retina, termed *snowbanking* (Fig. 2). This is best visualized by 20D indirect ophthalmoscopy, and indentation is required to exclude its presence.

Retinal Vasculitis

There are many features of vascular changes in PSII, and not all embody the overarching term *retinal vasculitis*. Additionally, there is little evidence to support the term retinal vasculitis in terms of inflammation of the vessel pathologically as seen in biopsies of systemic vasculitides. Although we recognize that systemic vasculitis can present with intraocular inflammation, the *retinal vasculitis* we commonly observe clinically is a result of infiltrating retinal inflammatory cells creating a *perivascular cuff* or a result of vascular occlusion (Fig. 3). Retinal vasculitis is potentially *sight-threatening* and more frequently affects the retinal venules rather than arterioles. Retinal vasculitis may exist as a predominant sign in posterior uveitis, but is also seen in most other forms of PSII, including *intermediate uveitis* and in posterior uveitis such as *chorioretinitis* or in association with systemic disease (Table 4).

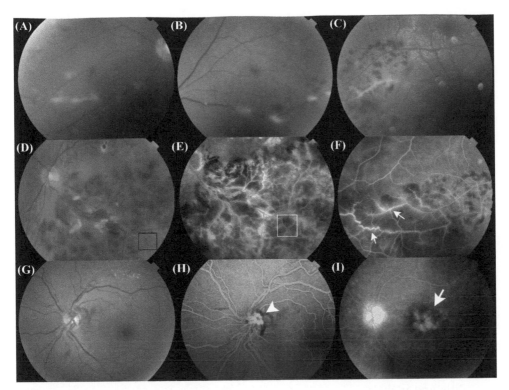

Figure 3 Fundus color photographs and fluorescein angiographs. (**A, B**) Venous sheathing or cuffing is a characteristic sign of retinal vasculitis. (**C, D**) Vasculitis may lead to closure of the lumen with resulting retinal swelling, hemorrhage, and cotton wool spots in the territory served by the affected vein. Fluorescein angiography may be used to demonstrate retinal ischemia (**D, E,** *boxed regions*), vessel wall staining and leakage (**F,** *arrow*), and cystoid macular edema (**I,** *arrow*). Neovascularization may also occur (**G, H,** *arrowheads*). *Source*: From Ref. Hughes EH, Dick AD. The pathology and pathogenesis of retinal vasculitis. *Neuropathology and Applied Neurobiology* (2003); 29:325–340.

Table 4 Causes and Associations of Retinal Vasculitis

Noninfectious associations	Infectious agents
Behçet's disease	*Mycobacterium tuberculosis*
Sarcoidosis	*Treponema pallidum*
Systemic lupus erythematosis	*Toxoplasma gondii*
Multiple sclerosis	*Bartonella henselae*
Seronegative arthropathies	*Borrelia burgdorferi*
Inflammatory bowel disease	*Brucella*
Sjogren's syndrome	*Leptospira*
Polyarteritis nodosa	HIV
Wegener's granulomatosis	HTLV1
Relapsing polychondritis	Herpesviridae—HSV, VZV, CMV, EBV
Lymphoproliferative disorders	
Drug-induced	

Source: Adapted from Ref. Hughes EH, Dick AD. The pathology and pathogenesis of retinal vasculitis. Neuropathol Appl Neurobiol 2003; 29:325–340.
Abbreviations: HSV, Herpes simplex virus; VZV, Varicella zoster virus; CMV, cytomegalovirus; EBV, Epstein-Barr virus.

Symptoms It is often asymptomatic, unless associated with panuveitis or intermediate uveitis, where floaters and loss of vision may occur more acutely. Symptoms of retinal vasculitis occur as a result of complications of retinal vasculitis and include

- loss of vision resulting from macular ischemia or vitreous hemorrhage secondary to retinal neovascularization,
- visual field loss as a result of vascular occlusion (vein or artery), and
- insidious visual loss as a result of venous stasis.

In one sample of 150 patients with PSII of predominant features of retinal vasculitis, 45% of cases have isolated ocular disease, and the remainder are associated with systemic inflammatory disorders. Of note was that two-thirds of patients were under 40 years of age, with a female preponderance. In most studies, the condition was notably bilateral in most cases, and the worse prognosis was seen in those cases with retinal ischemia as a result of retinal vascular occlusion.

In summary, *active retinal vasculitis* is observed with signs of

- retinal vessel engorgement and irregular dilatation,
- retinal vascular leakage—retinal edema, blurring of vascular margin, and then sheathing, and
- retinal vascular occlusion—leading to swelling, hemorrhages and exudates, and finally neovascularization.

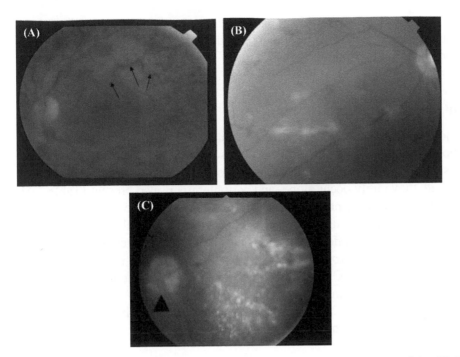

Figure 4 Composite fundus color photograph of patients with retinal vasculitis. (**A**) Posterior vasculitis presenting as venous stasis, showing tortuous vessels with irregular margins (*arrows*) and associated hemorrhages. (**B**) Peripheral vasculitis showing sheathed vessel. (**C**) Central vasculitis demonstrating blurred margins of optic nerve head (*arrowhead*) with capillary dilatation and central macular vasculitis with exudates.

Clinically, we can further define retinal vasculitis with respect to the fundal topography of retinal vascular involvement (Fig. 4).

- **Peripheral retinal vasculitis**—often low-grade and associated with blurring of vascular margins or sheathing of vessels with or without perivascular hemorrhage. Clinical assessment to distinguish between active and inactive vasculitis can be difficult. However, often when inactive, the sheathing is well-defined.
- **Posterior retinal vasculitis**—often presenting with occlusive disease with branch venous occlusion or venous stasis, with blurring of vessel margins, tortuous vessels, perivascular hemorrhages, and retinal swelling. Often results in chronic blood-ocular barrier breakdown and persistent cystoid macular edema.
- **Central retinal vasculitis**—where retinal vasculitis affects the optic nerve head or macular branches, resulting in disk swelling, venous and optic

nerve head capillary dilatation, and hemorrhage. However, frequently, unlike arteritic anterior ischemic optic neuropathies, it is unusual to elicit a relative afferent pupillary defect.

Arterial Vs. Venous Involvement

The majority of retinal vasculitis affects venules. This is seen predominantly in both idiopathic retinal vasculitis and most vasculitides associated with systemic disease such as sarcoidosis and multiple sclerosis. However, when the arterioles are involved, they rarely occur alone, and periphlebitis is also present (Table 5). It is also important to remember that retinal vasculitis, let alone arteritis, is rarely caused by systemic vasculitides such as Wegener's granulomatosis, Churg-Strauss, or polyarteritis nodosa. Infections are the more likely causes, principally the herpesviridae and *Toxoplasma*. When isolated vasculitis is associated with central nervous system (CNS) signs, then both Susac's syndrome (a micro-angiopathy of cochlea, retinal arteries, and CNS parenchyma) and antineutrophil cytoplasmic antibody (ANCA)-positive vasculopathies, or rarely Behçet's disease (see below for investigations and chap. 3) occur.

Evidence of Associated Choroidal Vasculopathy

Particularly in systemic-associated retinal vasculitis or systemic vasculitides that rarely present with intraocular inflammation, they may display choroidal involvement, in particular, choriocapillaris. While not obviously strictly a retinal vasculitis and one of the cardinal feature of PSII, it remains a significant feature

Table 5 Commoner Causes of Periphlebitis and Arteritis

Venulitis (periphlebitis)	Arteritis	Arteritis and periphlebitis
Intermediate uveitis	Susac's syndrome	Systemic vasculitides
Sarcoidosis	Systemic vasculitides[a] (ANCA-positive)	*Toxoplasma* chorioretinitis
Multiple sclerosis	Herpetic retinopathies	Syphilis
Inflammatory bowel disease	*Toxoplasma* chorioretinitis Syphilis	Tuberculosis—*Eale's disease*
Seronegative arthropathies		

[a]Systemic vasculitides include Churg-Strauss, Wegener's granulomatosis, polyarteritis nodosa, and ANCA-positive vasculitides.
Abbreviation: ANCA, antineutrophil cytoplasmic antibody.

of some of the posterior uveitides. Characteristically, this may not be identified unless there are associated pigment epithelial changes, without angiography (see below). Occlusive choriocapillaris disease is observed as a primary event in Systemic lupus erythematosus (SLE) and related anti-phospholipid syndromes and lymphoproliferative disease but also forms part of inflammation in white dot syndromes and acute posterior multifocal placoid pigment epitheliopathy (APMPPE), and awareness about other posterior uveitides is increasing.

In summary, retinal vasculitis is a descriptive term in which there is evidence of intraocular inflammation in the presence of predominant retinal vascular changes. As such we will not be discussing occlusive vasculopathies in the absence of any signs of inflammation such as anti-phospholipid syndromes.

When clinically assessing a patient for retinal vasculitis, the following are of particular note:

- Appearance of optic disc
- Involvement of arterioles, venules or capillaries or both
- Presence of hemorrhages and exudates (often signs of severe disease and/or occlusive disease)
- Presence of Retinal Pigment Epithelium (RPE)/choroidal involvement
- Associated structural changes—macular edema
- Associated neovascularization

Chorioretinitis

Chorioretinitis represents cellular infiltrates within the choroid and outer retina and can occur as single, multifocal, discrete small to large confluent lesions in many forms of posterior uveitis (chap. 3). More particularly, chorioretinitis is found associated with predominant vitritis in *intermediate uveitis* and also in *panuveitis* as well as milder, more chronic inflammatory conditions in which there is largely an absence of vitritis, the *white dot syndromes*. Their presence can be characteristic of both certain infectious and noninfectious conditions, but *beware*, there is considerable overlap.

Symptoms Classically their presence is associated with scintillation and, more rarely, photopsia. However, again, as we have discussed in relation to retinal vasculitis, symptoms may vary as to whether the chorioretinitis occurs as part of a more profound intraocular inflammation such as panuveitis.

In summary,

- when the choroiditis is either peripapillary or at the macula, then reduced vision may occur acutely,

- if insidious, at the onset of chorioretinitis, there may be symptoms relating to positive scotomata,
- metamorphopsia and blurring of central vision occur either because the choroiditis is at the macula or secondary to adjacent retinal edema, inflammation-induced choroidal neovascularization,
- in milder forms of chorioretinitis (*white dot syndromes*), there may be associated visual loss, which improves over several weeks, or signs of metamorphopsia/micropsia, which again resolve, and
- scotoma may occur as a result of associated enlarged blind spot in association with white dot syndromes.

Signs Chorioretinal lesions are very varied in their presentation. As you will see in chapter 3, some chorioretinal features and phenotype permit almost "specific" diagnoses to be recognized. However, chorioretinal lesions are obviously best visualized with indirect ophthalmoscopy, but remember

i. their features may vary throughout the course of disease
ii. there is considerable overlap and chorioretinal lesions are not always readily diagnostic (multifocal choroiditis, punctuate inner choroidopathy, ocular histoplasmosis).
iii. It is necessary to define activity to best appropriate immunosuppressive therapy where and when required.

Clinically, activity is defined by (Fig. 5)

- ill-defined margin of lesion (as opposed to discrete margins of inactive lesions),
- creamy appearance (as opposed to transparent inactive lesions),
- associated (and often mild) vitritis in posterior vitreous gel (or retrohyaloid space), and
- associated retinal edema.

Retinitis, even without vitritis or anterior segment inflammation, may be the only feature of overlying vasculitis. Retinitis is observed frequently in patients with infection, who are systemically immunocompromised (see below, Fig. 6, and chap. 3).

As part of the signs of PSII, chorioretinitis may of course coexist in patients with *posterior uveitis*, where both vitritis and retinal vasculitis are present (Fig. 7). Activity therefore can be noted and demonstrated by the appearance of chorioretinal lesion, retinal vasculitis, and the BIO vitreal haze score.

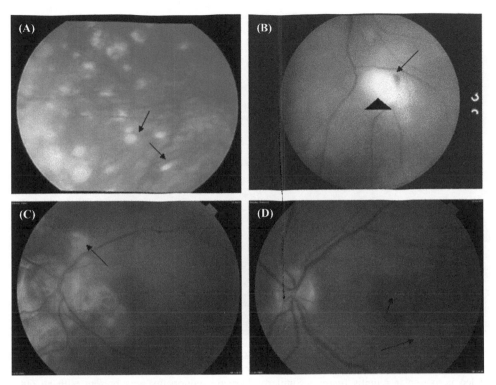

Figure 5   Composite fundus color photographs displaying spectrum of chorioretinitis. (**A**) Multifocal choroiditis. Active lesions, which are creamy and have indistinct margins (*arrows*). (**B**) Discrete unifocal lesion, which is again creamy and has indistinct margins (*arrowhead*) with associated hemorrhage (*arrow*), characteristic of a patient with *Toxoplasma chorioretinitis*. (**C**) Ill-defined edges of creamy confluent peripapillary lesions of serpiginous choroidopathy (*arrow*) (**D**) Small outer retinal/ choroidal lesions (*arrows*) of a patient presenting with scintillation and metamorphopsia due to multiple evanescent white dot syndrome (MEWDS).

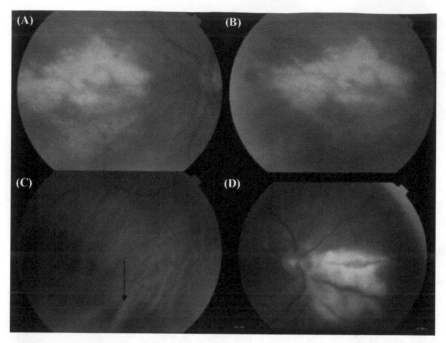

Figure 6 Composite fundus color photographs of retinitis. (**A, B**) Retinitis secondary to CMV retinitis in an immunocompromised bone marrow transplant patient. (**C**) Other areas of partially healed perivascular retinitis (*arrow*). Similarly, herpetic retinopathy may present with an outer retinal necrosis. (**D**) Varicella zoster–associated progressive outer retinal necrosis.

However, progressive choroidal lesions may present a diagnostic dilemma and should alert to the possibility of neither an infectious nor an autoinflammatory cause (Fig. 8).

Clinical Signs of Structural Changes Associated with PSII

The current consensus is that inflammation generates structural changes that are not specific for definition or characterization of the anatomical location of uveitis (*intermediate, posterior, or panuveitis*). Structural changes that should be assessed include

- retinal swelling/edema,
- cystoid macular edema,
- optic nerve head edema,
- retinal neovascularization,

- choroidal neovascularization,
- preretinal fibrosis—epiretinal membranes,
- subretinal fibrosis, and
- retinal breaks and associated rhegmatogenous retinal detachments.

Whether such clinical features form part of active inflammation or are indeed a consequence of resolved/treated inflammation can only be ascertained following full clinical assessment. The importance of determining activity in the presence of some of the structural changes highlighted above is to deliver correct management and treatment. To determine whether immunosuppressive therapy, for example, should continue or even be started is often difficult and, as we will highlight later, may lack substantial evidence for or against it. What is recognized is that any surgical intervention requires adequate immunosuppression to prevent relapse in PSII.

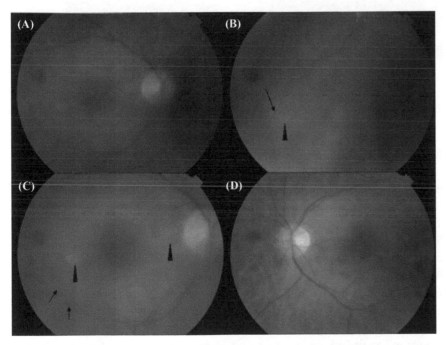

Figure 7 Composite fundus color photographs demonstrating a unilateral spectrum of signs in posterior segment intraocular inflammation. (**A**) Earlier in disease onset, BIO score is 2, with signs of both peripapillary and early posterior pole chorioretinitis. (**B, C**) Disease progression with increase in vitreal activity (BIO 3). Increased creamy and indistinct margins of chorioretinitis (*arrowheads*) with associated retinal vasculitis (*arrows*) in a patient with idiopathic disease. (**D**) Note that left eye is unaffected. *Abbreviation*: BIO, binocular indirect ophthalmoscopy.

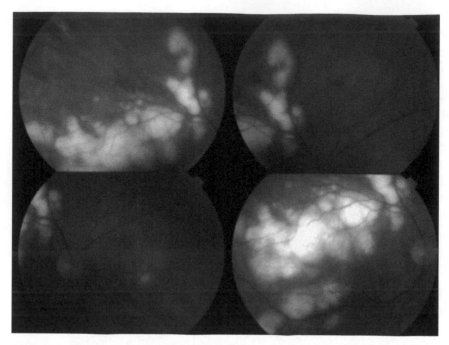

Figure 8 Composite fundus color photographs of patient with intraocular B-cell lymphoma. The composite photographs show both discrete and confluent choroidal lesions increasing over six weeks. Subsequent vitreous and lesional cytology confirmed the diagnosis of intraocular B-cell lymphoma.

DETERMINING INFECTIOUS VS. NONINFECTIOUS PSII

This issue when a patient presents to you, is whether his or her intraocular inflammation is infective or not. Obviously, this determines the best-directed treatment. While clearly, there is a large spectrum of infectious agents that may cause PSII, the likelihood of any one specific agent varies globally and is dependent on endemic status of organism and the immune constitution of the patient. All this becomes increasingly apparent with accurate history and systems inquiry. Clearly, as we will see in chapter 3, there are clinical features that direct our management toward investigations to establish which infection is responsible for intraocular inflammation while contemporaneously treating infection with a "broad spectrum" antiviral or antibacterial approach (Fig. 9). So overall, the paradigm to follow is to use clinical signs to determine whether the inflammation is infective or noninfective so that appropriate therapy can be instituted initially to provide the best chance to preserve vision. Changing treatments or reinvestigating is paramount once investigations and results flood in, but should not preclude starting treatment if the vision is threatened acutely.

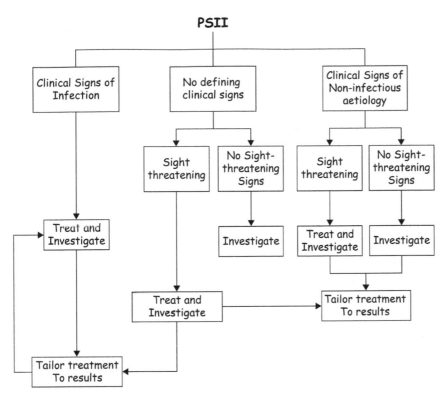

Figure 9 Generic algorithm for treatment of PSII. As you will discern in chapter 3, there are some features that make the diagnosis of infectious PSII very likely. The clinical features will therefore help in treating and investigating that patient appropriately. For the others, there may be no signs or history inquiry to highlight infection and therefore, the clinical decision for treatment should be based on sight-threatening features. Obviously, the treatments for infectious causes are microbe specific, and can be instituted generically as for presumed herpetic retinopathy or *toxoplasmosis* until investigations guide otherwise or further hone and tailor therapy accordingly. For treatment algorithm of sight-threatening noninfectious PSII, see fig. 10. *Abbreviation*: PSII, posterior segment intraocular inflammation.

DETERMINING SIGHT-THREATENING DISEASE

In terms of noninfectious PSII, one of the most important clinical decisions to make is whether or not there is presence of *sight-threatening disease*. Although we recognize that untreated PSII will lead to visual loss and, in the majority, will require immunosuppression of some form or the other [i.e., local versus systemic therapy (chaps. 4 and 5)] in the majority of cases, the decision as to whether there is a likelihood of acute visual loss or visual loss in the short term is paramount and will determine the extent of immunosuppressive therapy given initially, i.e., treating *sight-threatening* disease.

An accurate systemic workup as well as ocular signs will assist in determining sight-threatening disease. The issue becomes straightforward when the patient presents with visual loss either due to intense vitritis or chorioretinitis affecting the macular or retinal vasculitis. We also recognize that certain disorders have a higher prevalence of visual loss and a poorer long-term prognosis without treatment, which include Behçet's disease, Vogt-Koyanagi-Harada, central retinal vasculitis, and the more insidious birdshot chorioretinopathy and serpiginous choroiditis. Diagnosis of such cases is overviewed in chapter 3, engaging the international guidelines for diagnostic purposes.

Here we have developed a simple schema to assist in the treatment of patients with noninfectious PSII (Fig. 10). Treatment is often instituted at the same time with investigating patients for underlying systemic associations (see below), but is based on determining (*i*) whether PSII is noninfective and (*ii*) ocular signs of sight-threatening nature. These signs include

- significant vitritis (BIO grade of 3 or more),
- chorioretinitis affecting the posterior pole and macula,
- central retinal vasculitis (involvement of the optic nerve head),
- occlusive vasculitis, and
- neovascularization—retinal or choroidal.

To determine sight-threatening nature of PSII, ancillary imaging including fluorescein and indocyanine angiography, optical coherence tomography (OCT), and neuroimaging is frequently employed and directed following initial clinical assessment of patient (see below).

ASSESSING COEXISTING SYSTEMIC DISEASE IN PSII

Whether or not to have a blanket approach/screen in investigating patients is open to question. Given constraints on health care funding, most centers employ an iterative tailored approach in investigating underlying coexisting systemic

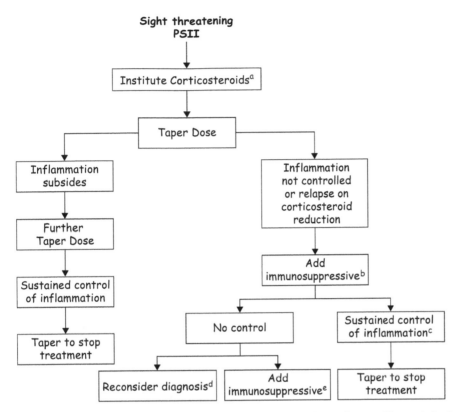

Figure 10 Generic algorithm for a suggested scheme for patients with noninfectious PSII. [a]Corticosteroid therapy—either oral (1–1.5 mg/kg/day) or intravenous (1 g/day for 3 days). Regimes vary depending on centers. [b]Additional immunosuppressives are varied and will be covered in chapter 5. Commonly used immunosuppressives include methotrexate, cyclosporine A, azathioprine, and more recently, tacrolimus and cellcept (mycophenolate mofetil). [c]With disease control, there should be drug-maintained remission for a minimum of six to nine months prior to further tapering of therapy. [d]If disease is difficult to control, then reconsider diagnosis of either underlying lymphoproliferative disease or infection (chronic herpetic retinopathy or ocular tuberculosis for example). [e]Some cases of PSII require "triple" immunosuppression by the addition of another agent (e.g., corticosteroids, cellcept, and tacrolimus). More recently, "biologic" therapy (anti-TNF and alpha-interferon therapy) has been instituted at this stage or even earlier in severe cases such as Behçet's disease with associated occlusive retinal vasculitis (chap. 5). *Abbreviation*: PSII, posterior segment intraocular inflammation. *Source*: Adapted from Ref. 4.

disease. There are some important points to make. First, the investigations of choice vary globally, depending on the prevalence of causes of uveitis in the area of investigation—particularly with relation to infectious PSII; second, the investigations should be tailored only after full ocular and systemic assessment of the patient, which will assist in directing your investigations.

General Investigations

- Blood pressure and urinalysis
- Full blood count and differential blood count
- Glucose
- Acute phase responses (such as plasma viscosity, erythrocyte sedimentation rate (ESR), or C-reactive protein)
- Liver function tests
- Creatinine and estimated glomerular filtration rate (eGFR)
- Cholesterol (lipid profile)
- Chest X ray

These tests form background to *baseline* assessment prior to immunosuppressive therapy as well as assessing underlying systemic disease when looking for indicators of systemic immune activation with raised acute-phase responses and abnormal liver function tests or presence of systemic vasculitis (rare), raised blood pressure, proteinuria or microscopic hematuria, glycosuria, raised creatinine, and reduced eGFR.

Tailored Investigations

- Serum angiotensin converting enzyme (ACE)
- Immune profile—antinuclear antibodies (dsDNA), anticardiolipin, lupus anticoagulant, ANCA including ELISA for anti-myeloperoxidase and anti Proteinase 3 (PR3) (polyarteritis nodosa and Wegener's granulomatosis, respectively)
- Infectious—HIV, VDRL (venereal disease research laboratory) or Fluorescent Treponemal antibody (FTA) for syphilis, mantoux or TB interferon-γ (IFNγ) Elispot, ELISA for *Borrelia* or *Bartonella*
- Ocular fluid sampling for polymerase chain reaction (PCR) for herpesviruses, *Toxoplasma*, IL-10 levels (lymphoma) or immunophenotyping and cytology
- Genetic studies [e.g., HLA (human leukocyte antigen)-B51 status and Behçet's disease, HLA-B27 and seronegative arthropathies]
- Lumbar puncture studies

Tailored investigations are also governed by the institution and vary globally, so different regions/countries employ different tests to screen, and therefore, the following is only a guide.

Tuberculosis   Though screening for TB varies globally, in general, a mantoux test (intradermal tuberculin) is employed if a patient is not already on immunosuppression, otherwise, results are inaccurate because of immunosuppression-mediated anergy. 48 to 72 hours after injection, a measurement of 6 to 15 mm suggests previous exposure (including environmental mycobacterium) or prior Bacillus Calmette-Guérin (BCG) vaccination and that greater than 15 mm is indicative of active mycobacterium tuberculosis exposure. The interpretation depends, however, on the risk, so in patients from endemic areas or high-risk occupational groups, a reading of greater than 6 mm may indicate infection. Also, HIV and immunosuppression or recent viral infections can produce a false-negative result. The more recent IFNγ Elispot may be beneficial as it is more sensitive and not as influenced by prior BCG vaccination or concurrent immunosuppression.

Syphilis   Syphilis detection tests vary between laboratories. In the majority, the tests used may include VDRL, TPHA (*Treponema pallidum* hemagglutination assay), RPR (rapid plasma reagin test), and FTA-ABS (flourescent treponemal antibody absorption).

HIV   Screening and diagnosis are tightly governed by most countries' department of health guidelines and should be referred to.

Lumbar puncture   Following neuroimaging (see below), particularly in suspected cases of CNS-related uveitis conditions, lumbar puncture is indicated. This will help determine extent of involvement and assist in diagnosis of multiple sclerosis, Vogt-Koyanagi-Harada, neurosarcoid or oculocerebral lymphoma. Of note, the opening cerebral spinal fluid (CSF) pressure (contributing to idiopathic intracranial hypertension) as well as measurement of protein, cells (pleocytosis/lymphocytosis), and presence of oligoclonal bands should be noted (Table 6).

Ocular fluid sampling   Both aqueous (aspiration) and vitreous sampling (including formal vitrectomy) are important tools to determine diagnosis. When diagnosis is indicative of herpes infection, PCR analysis of either aqueous or vitreous may confirm the diagnosis and tailor more specific antiviral therapy. Similarly, in cases of suspected intraocular lymphoma, initial aqueous sampling to demonstrate raised IL-10 levels may serve as a useful screen (5). More formal vitreous sampling is required to confirm diagnosis for immunophenotyping, cytology, and PCR molecular analysis.

Table 6 Commoner Causes of Pleocytosis and Oligoclonal Bands in CSF

Conditions	Pleocytosis[a]	Oligoclonal bands[b]
Multiple sclerosis	+/−	++
Behçet's disease	++	+
Sarcoidosis	++	+
Vasculitis (including SLE)	++	+
Vogt-Koyanagi-Harada	++	+/−
Oculocerebral lymphoma	+	+
Infectious		
Borellia	++	+
Treponema	++	+

[a]Pleocytosis refers to an increase in cell numbers, which is largely lymphocytosis in noninfectious PSII.
[b]Oligoclonal bands are bands of immunoglobulin (IgG), which are found in both CSF and serum. Paired sample is required to observe if its presence in cerebrospinal fluid (CSF), is specific and not just secondary to blood-brain barrier breakdown. Normally, two to five bands are considered significant. Interpretation of CSF oligoclonal bands in isolation is meaningless.
++ indicates high prevalence of oligoclonal bands or pleocytosis.

Tailored Imaging

- High-resolution spiral CT of chest
- MRI neuroimaging
- Neuroangiography or systemic angiography in cases of suspected systemic vasculitis

Most ancillary systemic investigations are performed in consort with guidance from intern.

Sarcoidosis The presence of raised ACE alone is not a sensitive predictor of sarcoidosis without either chest X-ray changes (e.g., bihilar lymphadenopathy) or confirmation by high-resolution spiral CT. Tissue diagnosis confirms diagnosis of sarcoidosis, and may be acquired via bronchoscopy or mediastinoscopic approach for lymph node biopsy if no other systemic features (e.g., peripheral lymphadenopathy or skin or conjunctival nodules) are more easily accessible for biopsy. Gallium scans are expensive but if positive with accompanying raised serum ACE, then are 98% specific for diagnosis.

Systemic vasculitis Remember this is a rare cause of PSII and retinal vasculitis. However, if clinical findings point toward the diagnosis (e.g., raised blood pressure, chest X-ray changes, proteinuria, and hematuria), further investigations are warranted. Backed by serological evidence (e.g., ANCA-positive), these warrant referral to appropriate intern for possible mesenteric angiography, neuroimaging, and renal or lung biopsy to ascertain diagnosis. Patients with vasculitis and no evidence of associated systemic inflammatory disease have increased morbidity for premature vascular disease (cerebral and cardiac). Therefore, ancillary investigations may also include factor V leiden, homocysteine, proteins C and S, and antithrombin 3 if predominant venous occlusive disease is present.

UTILIZING OCULAR IMAGING IN THE MANAGEMENT OF NONINFECTIOUS PSII

Frequently, despite accurate clinical assessment, the extent and severity of ocular inflammation and the degree of structural damage are gauged by an advantage of easy access and imaging of the retinal vasculature and tissue. These ancillary investigations are important to clearly define *sight-threatening* disease when there is doubt and also as a baseline to monitor therapeutic response and efficacy.

Angiography

Commonly employed are fluorescein angiography (FA) and indocyanine green angiography (ICGA). This enables the clinician to view with both FA and ICGA both the retinal and choroidal circulation, respectively. Fluorescein leaks readily from damaged (inflamed) retinal vessels and, conversely, will not flow through occluded vasculature. As a result, we are able to pick up with relative sensitivity

- early perivascular extravasation related to retinal vasculitis,
- retinal edema (in particular, cystoid macular edema), and
- areas of retinal ischemia as a result of occlusion.

Conversely, indocyanine green (ICG), which has a high-affinity binding to lipoproteins and is of larger molecular weight compared to FA, does not leak readily from vasculature. In the choroid, ICG will leak slowly from the fenestrated vessels, and with time, more ICG becomes sequestered into the choroidal stroma. The other advantage facilitating imaging of the choroid is that ICG fluoresces in the infrared (830 nm) range, allowing visualization through the retinal pigment epithelium. Therefore, with ICGA one can illustrate

- stromal choroidal disease and
- poor perfusion of the choriocapillaris.

Unlike FA, which observes most retinal vascular changes within five minutes of administration, ICG angiographic findings are elicited in three stages: *early phase* over first three minutes (demonstrating choriocapillaris and extravasations of dye into stroma), *intermediate phase* at 10 minutes (to show maximum choroidal stromal fluorescence), and finally, *late phase* at 25 to 30 minutes (to show wash-out of dye from choroidal vessels).

FLUORESCEIN ANGIOGRAPHY

Decision to undertake FA angiography is tailored for clinical need to elicit clinical suspicions of retinal vasculitis and to document the extent of disease, observe any vascular occlusive events, demonstrate vascular leakage and in particular (*i*) leakage at optic nerve head and/or cystoid macular edema and (*ii*) retinal and choroidal neovascularization. The following figures are examples of use of fluorescein angiography to demonstrate structural damage (cystoid macular edema) and evidence of *sight-threatening* disease (Figs. 11–15).

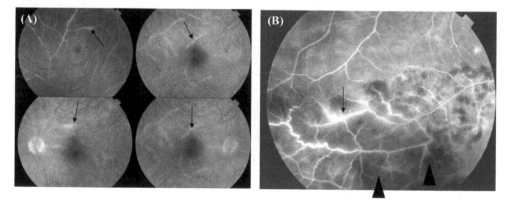

Figure 11 Fundus fluorescein angiography in patients with retinal vasculitis. (**A**) Composite angiographic evidence of retinal vasculitis (*arrows*) in patient with intermediate uveitis and no clinical central retinal signs. Note that vasculitis affects the posterior pole indicative of sight-threatening disease. (**B**) More aggressive retinal vasculitis with perivascular cuffing (fluorescein leakage, *arrow*) and areas of ischemia (non-perfusion, *arrowheads*). Both panels display signs of sight-threatening disease.

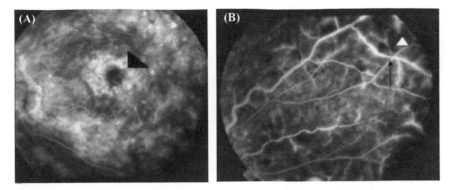

Figure 12 Fundus fluorescein angiography demonstrating active retinal vasculitis, ischemia, and cystoid macular edema in intermediate uveitis. (**A**) Fluorescein-angiographic appearance of cystoid macular edema (*black arrowhead*). (**B**) Peripheral retinal vasculitis (*arrow*) and non-perfusion (ischemia; *arrowhead*). Both features demonstrate sigh-threatening signs.

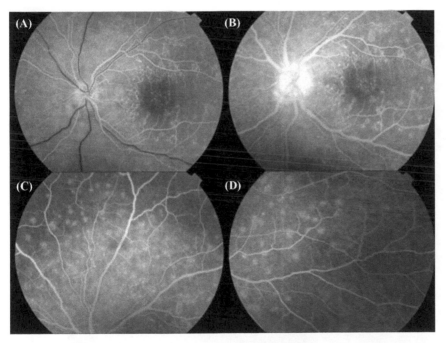

Figure 13 Fundus fluorescein angiography demonstrating extent of multifocal choroidal lesions early in evolution of birdshot choroidopathy. (**A–D**) Outer retinal/choroidal lesions in all phases of angiogram. Initially, they stain lightly (sometimes hypoflourescent), but as angiogram progresses, the stain increases. Such signs should not be taken in isolation, as they can be seen in most forms of white dot syndromes, multifocal choroiditis, and earliest stages of sympathetic ophthalmia, Vogt-Koyanagi-Harada, and birdshot retinochoroidopathy.

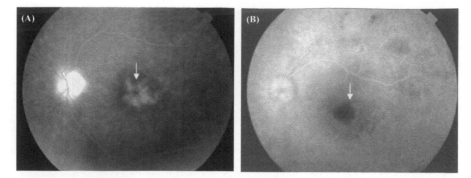

Figure 14 Fundus fluorescein angiography of patients with structural sequelae of intermediate uveitis. (**A**) Cystoid macular edema (*arrow*), which is most common feature of structural changes associated with posterior segment intraocular inflammation and leading to visual loss. However, as (**B**) shows, unrecognized retinal vasculitis in patient with intermediate uveitis can also lead to enlarged foveal avascular zone (*arrow*) secondary to ischemia.

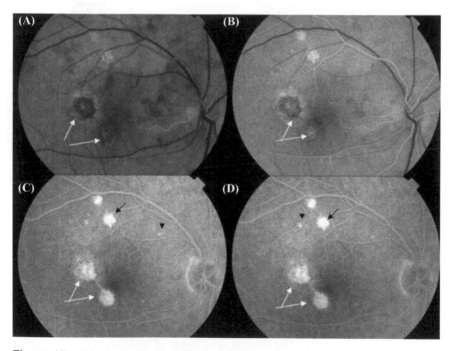

Figure 15 Sight-threatening complication of low-grade noninfectious posterior segment intraocular inflammation. The composite fundus FA demonstrates in a patient with punctuate inner choroidopathy (see chap. 3, page 114) the development of CNV. (**A**, **B**) Delineation of type II choroidal neovascularization. (**C**, **D**) Staining and minimal leakage from the CNV later in FA (*white arrows*) and also staining of other CNV. Extrafoveal (*arrows*) and choroidal inflammatory lesions (*arrowhead*). *Abbreviations*: FA, fluorescein angiography; CNV, choroidal neovascular membranes.

INDOCYANINE GREEN ANGIOGRAPHY

ICG angiography is increasingly used for demonstrating the extent of choroidal involvement in choroidal stromal pathologies (choroiditis) as well as white dot syndromes. ICG hypofluorescence is as a result of (*i*) non-perfusion during early stages in choriocapillaris and (*ii*) stromal disease (cellular infiltrate, granuloma), excluding extravasation of ICG into the stroma (6). There are attempts to reclassify disease according to ICG angiographic findings. However, without contemporaneous histology or animal model support, it is not possible to accurately correlate the two. Nevertheless, for the general management of patients with PSII, predominantly a posterior uveitis, the issue is to be able to define the extent of disease and therefore assist in indicating whether it is incipiently *sight threatening* or not. Hyperfluorescence, similar to its fluorescein counterpart, demonstrates leakage from inflamed vessels, optic nerve head, choroidal neovascular membrane, or granulomata. The following figures demonstrate the use of ICG angiography in PSII (Figs. 16–19).

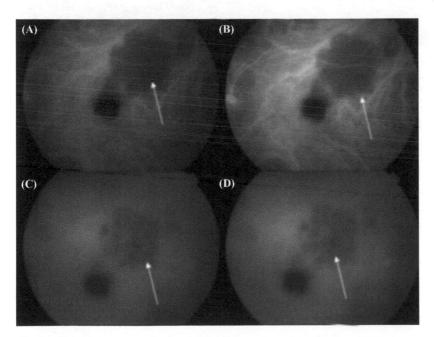

Figure 16 ICG angiography demonstrating persistent hypofluorescence in a patient with sarcoid granuloma. (**A–D**) Phases of ICG angiography. Arrow in all captions demonstrates that one of the lesions that excludes ICG throughout the angiogram. *Abbreviation*: ICG, indocyanine green.

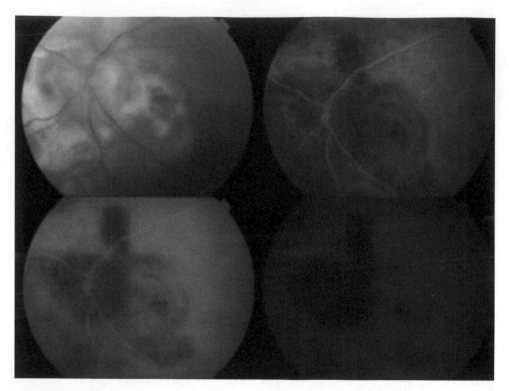

Figure 17 ICG angiography of patient with serpiginous choroidopathy. As compared with color fundus photograph, throughout the phases of ICG angiogram, there is persistent hypofluorescence and exclusion of ICG from stromal/choroidal lesion in characteristic peripapillary extension of disease observed clinically. *Abbreviation*: ICG, indocyanine green.

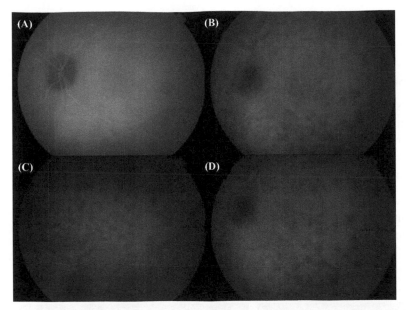

Figure 18 Composite ICG angiography in patient with MEWDS. (**A–D**) In late phase, persistence of hypoflourescent dots in patient with MEWDS. There were, as classically described, many more lesions than observed clinically. ICG can be used to demonstrate resolution or progression into multifocal choroiditis prior to clinical signs, and therefore allow early and appropriate immunosuppressive treatment. The features, however, should not be interpreted in isolation as they are not specific to MEWDS, and are observed in any "granulomatous" posterior uveitis. *Abbreviations*: ICG, indocyanine green; MEWDS, multiple evanescent white dot syndrome.

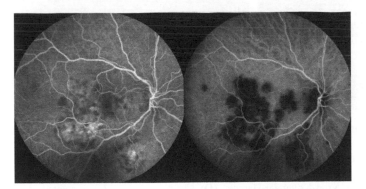

Figure 19 The benefits of combined fluorescein angiography and indocyanine green angiography. This figure demonstrates possible benefit of combined angiography. Fluorescein angiography shows lesions with areas of hypo- and hyperfluorescence (*right*), which may be seen with most cases of posterior uveitis associated with choroiditis. On the other hand, ICG angiography shows the dramatic early exclusion of ICG from choriocapillaris in a patient with acute posterior multifocal placoid pigment epitheliopathy (*left*). Again, however, in isolation, these examinations do not generate a diagnosis. Such findings can be observed in patients with serpiginous choroiditis or in infective posterior segment intraocular inflammation due to syphilis and tuberculosis. *Abbreviation:* ICG, indocyanine green.

Optical Coherence Tomography

With increasing resolution and speed of image acquisition, OCT is becoming a valuable noninvasive tool for the management of patients with PSII since one of the original descriptions of its use in uveitis (7). Its value is particularly in

- demonstrating, both topographically and quantitatively, macular disease,
- monitoring response of therapy for macular edema,
- monitoring response of therapy for choroidal neovascular membranes, and
- demonstrating secondary structural changes of epiretinal membranes and macular holes.

The following figures give examples of the use of OCT. In future, with ever increasing resolutions, we will also be able to assess cellular structural changes and predict outcomes and response to therapy (Figs. 20–22).

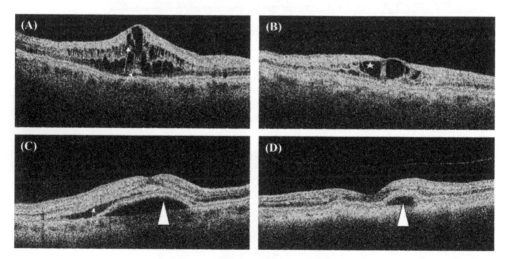

Figure 20 OCT demonstration of structural changes in PSII. This composite depicts the usefulness of OCT in demonstrating structural changes in patients with PSII. (**A, B**) Different intensities of cystoid macular edema with stretching of retinal glia (*arrow*) and deep retinal deposit (*arrow*) showing intraretinal pockets of fluid (*). (**C**) Intraretinal fluid (*arrow*) and subretinal fluid (*arrowhead*) in patient with Vogt-Koyanagi-Harada. (**D**) Fluid (*arrowhead*) associated with choroidal neovascular membrane in patient with punctuate inner choroidopathy. *Abbreviations:* OCT, optical coherence tomography; PSII, posterior segment intraocular inflammation.

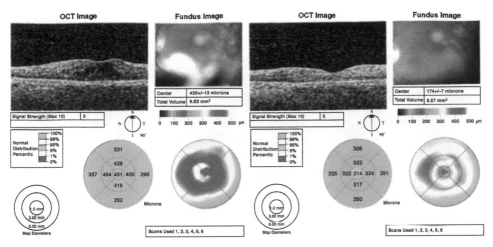

Figure 21 Documenting resolution of cystoid macular edema. OCT can document thickness maps and foveal height in patient with cystoid macular edema (CME) association with posterior segment intraocular inflammation. Treatment efficacy can be accurately monitored this way, as observed in this case, with a reduction in foveal thickness from 435 to 174 μm following treatment. *Abbreviation:* OCT, Optical coherence tomography.

UTILIZING VISUAL FUNCTION TESTS IN THE MANAGEMENT OF NONINFECTIOUS PSII

Both visual field testing and electrodiagnostic tests are very useful adjuncts in the management of PSII, and should be thought of in respect to

- establishing the extent of visual field loss on presentation in patients,
- documenting extent of damage from macular and optic nerve disease (scotoma size),
- establishing baseline retinal function at presentation,
- establishing cause of visual loss in PSII (retinal vs. optic nerve),
- monitoring response to treatment when clinical signs of activity are subtle (in, for example, birdshot chorioretinopathy), and
- assisting in firming the diagnosis in rare cases of PSII [acute zonal occult outer retinopathy (AZOOR) and autoimmune retinopathies] (8).

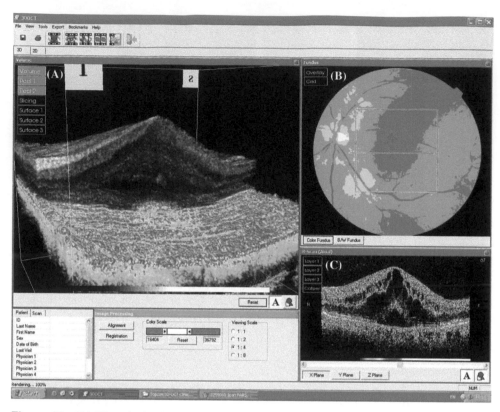

Figure 22 (**A**) 3D optical coherence tomography. This figure shows how volumetric assessment of patients with posterior segment intraocular inflammation and cystoid macular edema is enhanced by monitoring using 3D optical coherence tomography. (**B**) Representation of where OCT map was made from fundus image, and (**C**) standard OCT image.

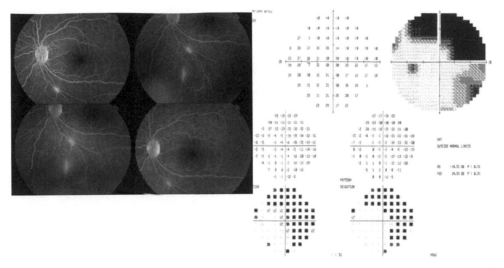

Figure 23 Visual fields to demonstrate loss of visual function. A fundus fluorescein angiogram of a patient with focal retinal arteritis associated with Susac's syndrome (retinocochleovestibular arteriopathy) (*right caption*). The affect on the retina, which was not apparent clinically, is demonstrated by marked field loss in the affected eye (*left caption*). Field loss fluctuated with immunosuppression in this patient, and thus, fields were used to document response to therapy.

Field testing, either with Goldmann field examination or with automated kinetic perimetry, assists documenting the extent of scotoma, particularly when macula or optic nerve is involved (such as in sarcoid, central vasculitis, or inflammatory optic neuropathies, as well as clinical entities such as enlarged big blind spot syndrome associated with white dot syndromes). It is important to document fields in all cases where there is clinical indication of CNS involvement. With electrodiagnostics, assessment of diminished visual function can be usefully monitored in chronic posterior uveitis, where clinical signs of activity are not always apparent (9).

REFERENCES

1. Jabs DA, Nussenblatt RB, Rosenbaum JT. Standardization of uveitis nomenclature for reporting clinical data. Results of the First International Workshop. Am J Ophthalmol 2005; 140(3):509–516.

2. Nussenblatt RB, Palestine AG, Chan CC, et al. Standardization of vitreal inflammatory activity in intermediate and posterior uveitis. Ophthalmology 1985; 92(4):467–471.

3. Chylack LT Jr., Wolfe JK, Singer DM, et al. The Lens opacities classification system III. The Longitudinal Study of Cataract Study Group. Arch Ophthalmol 1993; 111(6):831–836.

4. Jabs DA, Rosenbaum JT. Guidelines for the use of immunosuppressive drugs in patients with ocular inflammatory disorders: recommendations of an expert panel. Am J Ophthalmol 2001; 131(5):679.

5. Cassoux N, Giron A, Bodaghi B, et al. IL-10 measurement in aqueous humor for screening patients with suspicion of primary intraocular lymphoma. Invest Ophthalmol Vis Sci 2007; 48(7):3253–3259.

6. Cimino L, Auer C, Herbort CP. Sensitivity of indocyanine green angiography for the follow-up of active inflammatory choriocapillaropathies. Ocul Immunol Inflamm 2000; 8(4):275–283.

7. Antcliff RJ, Stanford MR, Chauhan DS, et al. Comparison between optical coherence tomography and fundus fluorescein angiography for the detection of cystoid macular edema in patients with uveitis. Ophthalmology 2000; 107(3): 593–599.

8. Francis PJ, Marinescu A, Fitzke FW, et al. Acute zonal occult outer retinopathy: toward a set of diagnostic criteria. Br J Ophthalmol 2005; 89(1):70–73.

9. Holder GE, Robson AG, Pavesio C, et al. Electrophysiological characterisation and monitoring in the management of birdshot chorioretinopathy. Br J Ophthalmol 2005; 89(6):709–718.

3

Practical Evaluation of the Patient in the Clinic

When one is faced with a patient having posterior segment intraocular inflammation (PSII) for the first time, the process of generating a list of differential diagnoses depends greatly on the predominant ocular signs or features. Although most diseases present with a degree of many features of inflammation, such as vitritis, retinal vasculitis, and/or choroiditis, there are often one or two features that predominate over the others. For example, retinal vasculitis may be the predominating feature in an eye that also has some vitritis and some papillitis. Retinal vasculitis as the predominant feature would lead us to consider the more likely diagnoses of Behçet's disease, sarcoidosis, and tuberculosis rather than other diseases. In this manner, distilling all the ocular signs into only one or two predominant clinical features can greatly aid in narrowing down the differential diagnosis. Of course, the differential diagnosis should also be tailored to other clinical characteristics of the patient's history and ocular examination, in particular, whether or not anterior segment inflammation is present.

Chapter 2 has already defined and offered hints on how to describe the major posterior uveitic features of vitritis, retinal vasculitis, and chorioretinitis. While this establishes the diagnosis of uveitis and its classification, and indeed recognizes sight-threatening lesions (further discussed in chap. 4), this chapter gives a concrete framework for the reader to generate differential diagnoses based on these and other predominant ocular features. Again, it should be emphasized that all ocular features should be graded and reported according to the Standardization of Uveitis Nomenclature (SUN) guidelines (1). The decision to begin treatment is not based on specific diagnosis but on deciding infective (where then a specific diagnosis of infective agent is imperative) or noninfective etiology, and whether immediately sight threatening or not. The descriptions within this chapter will help achieve this.

Nevertheless, making a diagnosis in noninfectious cases is important for determining long-term outcome and appropriate choices, where necessary, of immunosuppressive therapy.

DIFFERENTIAL DIAGNOSIS BASED ON PREDOMINANT OCULAR FEATURE

The following is an outline of the *most likely* candidates for specific disease entities based on the *predominant* posterior segment feature. As you might expect, there is overlap of clinical signs among many of the conditions since the ocular tissues have a limited set of responses to injury, but the key to diagnosis often lies in the pattern of signs as they develop both in time and space. The lists are subdivided based on additional characteristics, such as whether *significant* (1+ or greater) vitritis and/or anterior segment inflammation accompanies the predominant feature (Fig. 1). Infectious diseases are listed first followed by noninfectious

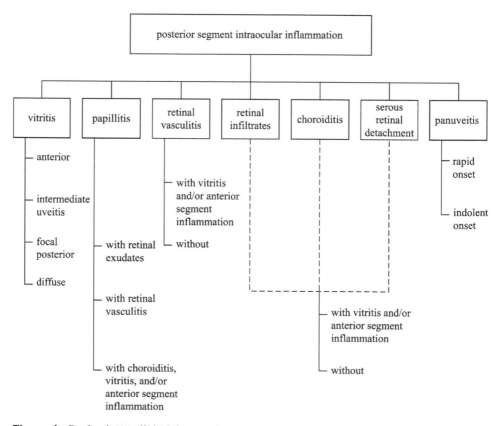

Figure 1 Predominant clinical features in posterior segment intraocular inflammation.

disorders and, where appropriate, the neoplastic disease intraocular lymphoma. Diseases that can present with many different predominant features appear in several sections, which only emphasizes the spectrum of phenotype each diagnosis may include and why treatment decisions cannot be based on making a diagnosis alone. Finally, a section on panuveitis in which the predominant feature *is* the presence or development of both posterior and anterior segment inflammation is also included. Rare diseases or ill-defined entities and rare presentations of common diseases are not included. Nonspecific features of chronic inflammation, such as *cystoid macular edema* and *epiretinal membrane*, are also left out of these differential diagnosis lists because they can occur in virtually any type of intraocular inflammation. Finally, the lists pertain mainly to clinical settings in developed countries worldwide. Diseases of the developing world, most notably tropical infections, as well as rare diseases are included in the second half of this chapter describing the workup for specific disease entities.

Vitritis

Some degree of vitritis is a feature of many diseases with PSII. But if vitritis is the *predominant* feature, the disorder is often classified as *intermediate uveitis*, and certain conditions and diseases, listed below, may present with it. The purpose of this chapter is to emphasize that while classifying the patient anatomically (e.g., intermediate vs. posterior vs. panuveitis), characteristics of the vitritis may assist in diagnosis of specific conditions, particularly in differentiating infective versus noninfective causes. For example, in general, acute or episodic vitritis would hint toward bacterial endophthalmitis (in a painful red eye), toxoplasmosis (with a chorioretinal scar present) (Fig. 2), or noninfectious PSII such as Behçet's

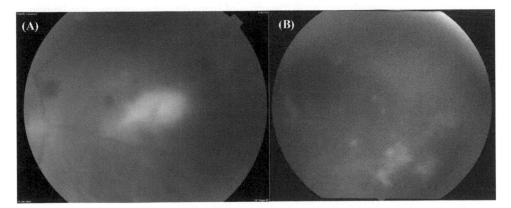

Figure 2 What can underlie a vitritis? (**A**) Characteristic *Toxoplasma* chorioretinal lesion with vitritis. (**B**) Numerous snowball-like opacities in the inferior vitreous in a patient with sarcoidosis.

disease (history of painful oral ulcers, and skin or genital lesions), whereas a chronic or indolent vitritis would suggest diseases such as sarcoidosis (often no systemic symptoms), malignant lymphoma (patient more than 50 years of age), and fungal endophthalmitis (recent hospitalization or surgery). Furthermore, chronic vitritis with snowball-like clumps inferiorly is characteristic of sarcoidosis (Fig. 2).

On the other hand, chronic vitritis just behind an intraocular lens with posterior capsular opacification is suspicious of delayed-onset postoperative endophthalmitis (particularly, *Propionibacterium acnes* infection after cataract surgery). The more typically ascribed *intermediate uveitis* is considered in a separate category below, since this classically and accurately represents a distinct clinical picture of chronic vitritis in the presence of exudates or snowbanking over the pars plana and/or peripheral retina, often accompanied by peripheral retinal vasculitis (see chap. 1). Looking in more detail at the anatomical distribution of inflammation, we can describe: "anterior vitritis" implying prominent vitreous cells centered behind the lens/iris diaphragm, observed best with the plain slit lamp, and "intermediate uveitis," "focal posterior vitritis" and "diffuse vitritis" best appreciated by contact lens biomicroscopy using the slit lamp or indirect ophthalmoscopy (Box 1).

Papillitis

As with vitritis, papillitis may be observed to some degree in any inflamed eye. However, it is the *predominant* feature in just a few diseases of PSII as listed below (Box 2), depending on accompanying ocular signs. An enlarged disc with prominent cellular infiltration may also represent a disc granuloma, suggestive of sarcoidosis (Fig. 3) or tuberculosis. Of course, papillitis or inflammation of the optic nerve head must always be differentiated from disorders of vascular ischemia (anterior ischemic optic neuropathy, giant cell arteritis, impending central retinal vein occlusion, diabetes mellitus), of acute demyelination (idiopathic optic neuritis), or of a genetic nature (Leber's hereditary optic neuropathy). These occur in eyes with no other evidence of intraocular inflammation in patients with characteristic medical or family history and are not included here. Finally, papillitis must be distinguished from papilledema, which occurs in disorders associated with increased intracranial pressure and would prompt an entirely different line of workup. Fluorescein angiography can be helpful here.

Retinal Vasculitis

Inflammation may predominantly involve retinal arteries or retinal veins. The classic teaching is that inflammation of retinal arteries is characteristic of diseases such as systemic lupus erythematosus and syphilis, while inflammation of retinal

---

Box 1 Conditions Causing a Predominant Vitritis

Anterior vitritis

- Delayed-onset postoperative endophthalmitis
- Toxocariasis

Intermediate uveitis with prominent vitritis

- Human T lymphocyte virus type 1 uveitis
- Lyme disease
- Syphilis
- Toxocariasis
- Sarcoidosis
- Multiple sclerosis
- Pars planitis
- Intraocular lymphoma

Focal posterior vitritis

- Fungal endophthalmitis
- Toxoplasmosis
- Toxocariasis

Diffuse vitritis

- Human T lymphocyte virus type 1 uveitis
- Bacterial endophthalmitis
- Lyme disease
- Fungal endophthalmitis
- Toxoplasmosis
- Toxocariasis
- Sarcoidosis
- Behçet's disease
- Immune recovery uveitis
- Intraocular lymphoma

---

veins is characteristic of diseases such as tuberculosis, sarcoidosis, and Behçet's disease. However, in practice, this distinction is of limited use since the division is far from foolproof, and most eyes show evidence of inflammation in both types of vessels. Signs suggestive of active retinal vasculitis (Fig. 4) include vascular

Box 2   Conditions Causing a Predominant Papillitis

With retinal exudates

- *Bartonella* infection (cat scratch disease, neuroretinitis)

With retinal vasculitis

- Toxoplasmosis
- Multiple sclerosis

With choroiditis, vitritis and/or anterior segment inflammation

- Tuberculosis
- Syphilis
- Vogt-Koyanagi-Harada disease
- Sarcoidosis

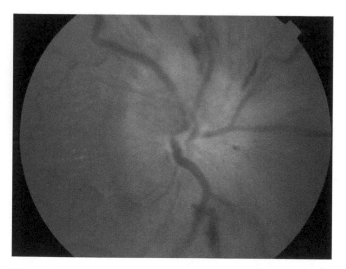

Figure 3 Fundus color photograph of swollen optic nerve head secondary to sarcoid granuloma.

tortuosity, dilation of retinal veins, and narrowing of retinal arteries. Active retinal vasculitis may be accompanied by varying degrees of retinal hemorrhage, perivascular cellular infiltrates, perivascular exudates, vitritis, posterior hyaloid traction over vessels, and/or cotton wool spots. The presence of cotton wool spots suggests retinal ischemia, and areas of retinal nonperfusion may be observed on

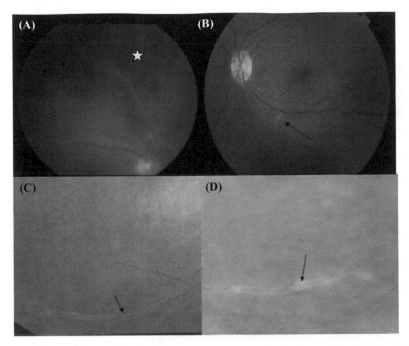

Figure 4 Fundus color photographs of features of retinal vasculitis. (**A**) Retinal hemorrhages (*) associated with retinal periphlebitis in a patient with tuberculosis. (**B**) Small occlusive vasculitis and cotton wool spot (*arrow*). (**C**) Prominent vascular sheathing (*arrow*) is seen in this patient with SLE being treated with immunosuppression. (**D**) Patient with retinal vasculitis shows the phenomenon of "cuffing" around vessels (*arrow*), representing active perivascular inflammation. (C and D reproduced with permission Bunkodo Publishing Company, Tokyo)

fluorescein angiography. Long-standing vascular ischemia may lead to neo-vascularization at the disc or in the retina. Well-demarcated sheathing of retinal vessels or ghost vessels (total occlusion) is indicative of chronic inflammation or inactive disease. Sheathing, which is irregular or patchy, and, importantly, produces a hazy, less well-defined "cuffing" around a segment of the vessel denotes active vasculitis.

Frosted branch angiitis is a particular form of retinal vasculitis associated with cytomegalovirus (CMV) and other infections. Although retinal vasculitis is a clinical feature observed in many disorders of intraocular inflammation, the list of diseases in which retinal vasculitis is the *predominant* feature is relatively short (Box 3).

Retinal Infiltrates

Cellular retinal infiltrates (retinitis) are the *predominant* feature in a surprisingly small number of disease entities, the overwhelming majority of which are

---

Box 3   Conditions Causing a Predominant Retinal Vasculitis

With significant vitritis and/or anterior segment inflammation

- Tuberculosis
- Behçet's disease
- Sarcoidosis

Without significant vitritis and/or anterior segment inflammation

- Whipple's disease
- Systemic lupus erythematosus
- Multiple sclerosis
- Frosted branch angiitis

Box 4   Conditions Causing a Predominant Retinal Infiltrate

With significant vitritis and/or anterior segment inflammation

- Acute retinal necrosis
- Bacterial endophthalmitis
- Fungal endophthalmitis
- Toxoplasmosis
- Behçet's disease

Without significant vitritis and/or anterior segment inflammation

- Cytomegalovirus retinitis
- Progressive outer retinal necrosis

---

infections (Box 4). With the exception of fungal endophthalmitis and CMV retinitis, all of the diseases have a rather acute onset, and except for CMV retinitis and progressive outer retinal necrosis (PORN), all are usually accompanied by a significant degree of vitritis and/or anterior segment inflammation. All of the infections are progressive in nature until specific antimicrobial treatment is initiated. The one noninfectious entity on the list, Behçet's disease, occurs in acute bursts of inflammation (Fig. 5) that are self-limiting but recurrent.

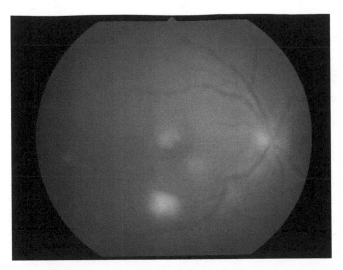

Figure 5 Fundus photograph of a typical posterior attack in a patient with Behçet's disease, showing several retinal infiltrates, disc hyperemia and edema, and engorgement of the vascular arcades. (With permission, Bunkodo Publishing Company, Tokyo)

Choroiditis (Choroidal White Dots and Other White Lesions)

White lesions in the choroid may appear in numerous intraocular inflammatory diseases, but are the hallmark of the diseases listed below (Box 5). Diseases commonly referred to as white dot syndromes (Fig. 6) include multifocal evanescent white dot syndrome (MEWDS), acute posterior multifocal placoid pigment epitheliopathy (APMPPE), and punctate inner choroidopathy (PIC). However, many textbooks include other diseases such as Vogt-Koyanagi-Harada (VKH) disease, and there is no definitive etiological, clinical, or anatomical reason for classifying one disease as "white dot disease" versus another disease as "multifocal choroiditis." Therefore, the following list ignores the designation of "white dot syndrome" and is divided in a more clinically relevant manner of whether significant vitritis and/or anterior segment inflammation accompanies the choroidal findings. Some diseases such as tuberculosis can present either with or without significant vitritis and/or anterior segment inflammation, and therefore appear in both sections of the list. Acute lesions tend to have indistinct borders, while old atrophic lesions have distinct borders often with pigmentation. Lesions that grow in size and coalesce may suggest acute retinal necrosis (ARN) due to herpes simplex virus (HSV) or varicella-zoster virus (VZV) infection (Fig. 7).

Many diseases that present with vitritis and/or anterior segment inflammation in the acute phase will only have atrophic choroidal lesions in the quiescent phase in absence of vitreous or anterior chamber cells. Therefore, one must

---

Box 5 Conditions Causing Predominant Choroidal White Lesions

With significant vitritis and/or anterior segment inflammation

- Acute retinal necrosis
- Tuberculosis
- Toxoplasmosis
- Toxocariasis
- Sarcoidosis
- Vogt-Koyanagi-Harada disease
- Sympathetic ophthalmia
- Multifocal choroiditis with panuveitis
- Birdshot choroidopathy
- Intraocular lymphoma

Without significant vitritis and/or anterior segment inflammation

- Tuberculosis
- Presumed ocular histoplasmosis and histoplasmosis-like disease
- Multifocal evanescent white dot syndrome
- Acute posterior multifocal placoid pigment epitheliopathy
- Punctate inner choroidopathy
- Serpiginous choroidopathy
- Intraocular lymphoma

---

always keep in mind the "phase" of the disease while examining the patient. In many conditions, the choroidal infiltrates begin near or actually extend from the optic disc (e.g., sarcoidosis, serpiginous choroidopathy, punctate inner choroiditis, and others) and as a result the normally circular optic nerve head can take on a "disfigured" or "moth-eaten" appearance (Fig. 8). In addition, this can produce an enlargement of the blind spot.

Serous Retinal Detachment

It is said that the hallmark of serous retinal detachment is the shifting nature of the subretinal fluid. However, small areas of serous retinal detachment, for example, confined to the posterior pole as seen in VKH disease (Fig. 9), will not shift. In all cases, a retinal break causing a rhegmatogenous retinal detachment or vitreous traction causing a tractional retinal detachment should be ruled out, as both can

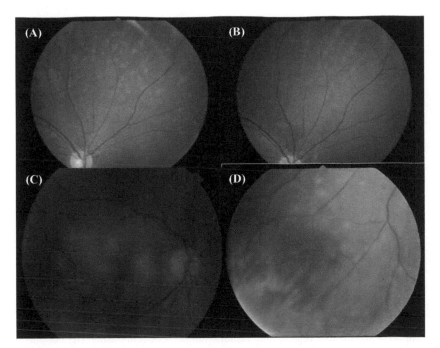

Figure 6 Composite fundus color photographs of various white dot syndromes. (**A**) Multiple white dots at the level of the RPE were observed in the peripheral retina of this patient diagnosed with multifocal evanescent white dot syndrome. (**B**) Six days later, most of the white dots were found to have resolved. (**C**) Patient with characteristic choriocapillaris/RPE lesions of APMPPE and (**D**) patient with Vogt-Koyanagi-Harada disease had a posterior recurrence of inflammation during tapering of systemic corticosteroids in the form of multifocal choroiditis. Note the multiple white spots that are deep to the retina, particularly toward the top of the photograph. These white spots resolved after an increase in the dose of corticosteroids. *Abbreviations*: RPE, retinal pigment epithelium; APMPPE, acute posterior multifocal placoid pigment epitheliopathy.

also occur as a complication in eyes with chronic inflammation, such as due to sarcoidosis. However, once the feature of serous retinal detachment is confirmed, one needs to consider only a few specific diseases, all of which are noninfective (Box 6). Uveal effusion syndrome, not an intraocular inflammatory disease, is included only for the purposes of listing the most likely candidates to consider in the differential diagnosis. Uveal effusion syndrome should be suspected if there is no vitritis and/or anterior segment inflammation and no choroidal leakage on fluorescein angiography, particularly if the eye is nanophthalmic. Serous retinal detachment due to inflammatory disorders is generally indicative of active choroidal inflammation and will generally exhibit some fluorescein leakage at the choroid or retinal pigment epithelium (RPE) level on angiography.

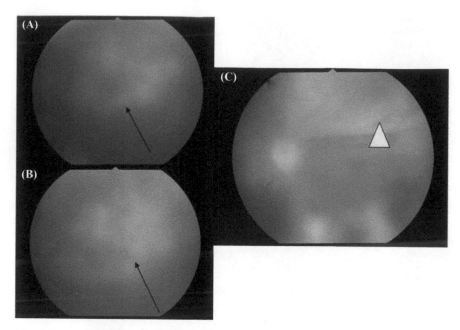

Figure 7 Fundal color photographs representing evolution of herpetic retinopathy. (**A**) Peripheral areas of retinal whitening (*arrow*) indicative of retinitis and/or retinal necrosis in a patient diagnosed with acute retinal necrosis due to the varicella-zoster virus. (**B**) Two days later, the involved area was noted to have increased in size (*arrow*). (**C**) Continuing necrosis may result in retinal detachment (*arrowhead*).

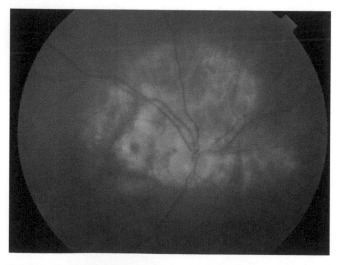

Figure 8 Fundus color photograph demonstrating peripapillary atrophy in a patient with serpiginous choroidopathy.

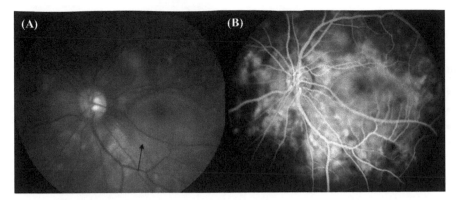

Figure 9   Serous retinal detachments in Vogt-Koyanagi-Harada disease. (**A**) Multifocal areas of serous retinal detachment are observed in the posterior pole in this patient with Vogt-Koyanagi-Harada disease (*arrow*). (**B**) Corresponding dye leakage and pooling is observed on fluorescein angiography.

Box 6   Conditions Causing Predominant Serous Retinal Detachments

With significant vitritis and/or anterior segment inflammation

- Vogt-Koyanagi-Harada disease
- Sympathetic ophthalmia
- Sarcoidosis

Without significant vitritis and/or anterior segment inflammation

- Posterior scleritis
- Systemic lupus erythematosus
- Uveal effusion syndrome

Panuveitis

When both significant anterior segment intraocular inflammation and significant PSII *are* the predominant features of a clinical presentation, the most likely diseases are fairly limited (Box 7). Of course, all of the diseases are also given on other lists above. This particular list is divided into diseases with rapid onset occurring over a few days versus those with more indolent onset of signs and symptoms occurring over weeks to months.

Box 7 Conditions Causing Panuveitis

Rapid onset (over days)

- Bacterial endophthalmitis
- Behçet's disease
- Vogt-Koyanagi-Harada disease
- Sympathetic ophthalmia

Indolent onset (over weeks to months)

- Tuberculosis
- Syphilis
- Lyme disease
- Sarcoidosis

DESCRIPTIONS AND WORKUP FOR SPECIFIC DISEASE ENTITIES

Once a list of differential diagnoses is determined based on the predominant feature(s), diagnoses on that list may be given higher or lower priority (or ruled out entirely) using additional information in the history, symptoms, review of systems, or anterior segment examination. This process is represented in the flow chart (Fig. 10). The clinician must then consider ancillary tests as appropriate for the particular patient to extract evidence that may support or refute a possible diagnosis. One should avoid a "shotgun" approach to diagnostic testing, as it leads to increased cost and morbidity for the patient as well as false-positive or incidentally positive results that often spark further rounds of testing of little or no clinical value. Furthermore, like the saying "the punishment should fit the crime," one should probably not embark upon expensive and tedious ancillary tests for an ocular inflammatory condition that is mild, particularly in the absence of systemic manifestations.

The following is a disease-specific guide to clinical features and basic workup of patients, divided into the traditional categories of infectious diseases (viral, bacterial, fungal, and parasitic), presumed autoinflammatory diseases (with systemic manifestations and without systemic manifestations), and neoplastic disease.

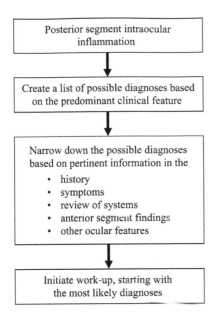

Figure 10 The thinking process prior to ordering ancillary tests.

Infectious Diseases: Viral

Viral infections, particularly the herpes family of viruses, have a particular propensity for infecting the retina. In this era of readily available polymerase chain reaction (PCR) testing, most causative viruses can be identified; however, treatment outcomes depend greatly on the immune status of the patient.

Acute Retinal Necrosis

ARN usually occurs in otherwise healthy individuals and can be caused by either one of the HSVs (type 1 or type 2) or the VZV. Since the clinical features are virtually indistinguishable for these viruses, accurate diagnosis is based on PCR of aqueous or vitreous humor (2). The standard treatment of intravenous acyclovir is generally effective for ARN in terms of halting progression of the retinitis, which usually starts in the periphery. Timely treatment will limit involvement of the optic nerve and macula, and one main determinant of visual outcome is whether optic atrophy and/or macular atrophy develop. The other main determinant of visual outcome is whether retinal detachment occurs as a secondary complication. The retinal detachment in ARN is rhegmatogenous and often develops within a few weeks of the onset of posterior vitreous detachment. Close monitoring of the vitreous may be helpful in alerting one to the possibility

Table 1 American Uveitis Society Criteria for the Diagnosis of ARN Syndrome

Criteria for use of the term "acute retinal necrosis syndrome"
1. One or more foci of retinal necrosis with discrete borders located in the peripheral retina
2. Rapid progression of disease if antiviral therapy has not been given
3. Circumferential spread of disease
4. Evidence of occlusive vasculopathy, with arteriolar involvement
5. Prominent inflammatory reaction in the vitreous and anterior chamber

Characteristics that support, but are not required for, a diagnosis of ARN syndrome
1. Optic neuropathy/atrophy
2. Scleritis
3. Pain

Abbreviation: ARN, acute retinal necrosis.
Source: From Ref. 5.

of incipient retinal detachment. To improve visual outcomes for this disease, some physicians advocate prophylactic vitrectomy with barrier laser photo-coagulation to the borders of healthy retina in eyes with significant vitreous inflammation but no retinal detachment. However, there are no randomized clinical trials as of yet to support such prophylactic surgery. Rarely a patient with ARN may have a history of herpetic encephalitis or recent cutaneous zoster, and ARN can occur in neonates. ARN can also occur in acquired immunodeficiency syndrome (AIDS) or other immunocompromised patients (e.g., patients on chronic systemic corticosteroids), and the disease may progress rapidly in these cases. ARN has been reported in rare instances to be due to CMV (3), and atypical toxoplasmosis may mimic ARN (4). The American Uveitis Society published a set of diagnostic criteria for ARN based solely on clinical characteristics and does not depend on identification of virus (Table 1) (5).

- Presenting symptoms: Pain, photophobia, decreased vision, floaters
- Medical history/demographic associations: History of a prodromal flu-like illness may be elicited, rarely a history of recent encephalitis or zoster
- Ocular signs: Starts in one eye, but may eventually involve both eyes in one-third of patients, usually within a few weeks. *Anterior*: Moderate-to-severe granulomatous anterior segment inflammation, intraocular pressure frequently elevated in early phase of disease. *Posterior*: Progressively worsening vitritis, whitish yellow spots coalescing to patches of retinitis/retinal necrosis starting in the periphery and progressing toward the posterior pole (Fig. 7), prominent vasculitis with hemorrhage, macular edema, papillitis, optic atrophy, rhegmatogenous retinal detachment

- Systemic signs: None
- Workup: PCR of aqueous or vitreous samples for HSV and VZV. If PCR is not available, Goldmann-Witmer coefficient may be calculated from intraocular antibody titers (6). Human immunodeficiency virus (HIV) testing should be considered
- Treatment: Intravenous acyclovir followed by oral acyclovir or oral valacyclovir. Aspirin and systemic corticosteroids may be considered. Vitrectomy with laser photocoagulation, with or without silicone oil or gas tamponade, is performed for rhegmatogenous retinal detachment. The utility of prophylactic surgery is unknown
- Prognosis: Varies depending on degree of posterior pole involvement and whether retinal detachment develops

Progressive Outer Retinal Necrosis

PORN is a relatively rare variant on VZV-associated retinal infection that starts in the outer retina, giving a distinct pattern of whitening of large geographic areas of retina with initially little or no retinal edema, retinal hemorrhage, or vitritis. PORN has a predilection for individuals on immunosuppression and advanced AIDS patients, a characteristic that may play a role in the distinctive manifestation and pathogenesis of VZV infection in these patients. PORN will progress rapidly to full thickness retinal necrosis and optic atrophy, with poor visual outcomes in most cases despite treatment. Unfortunately, PORN usually starts in one eye at first, but eventually both eyes are involved in 70% of cases (7). Although rare, PORN may also be caused by other herpes family viruses such as HSV (8).

- Presenting symptoms: Decreased vision
- Medical history/demographic associations: Immunosuppression, AIDS, rarely a history of cutaneous zoster
- Ocular signs: Bilateral in 70%. *Anterior*: Minimal-to-no anterior segment inflammation. *Posterior*: Minimal-to-no vitritis, progressively enlarging patches of retinal whitening in multifocal areas (Fig. 11), papillitis initially. Vitritis, vascular sheathing, vascular occlusion, optic atrophy, and rhegmatogenous retinal detachment may develop in later stages
- Systemic signs: None specific to PORN
- Workup: PCR of aqueous or vitreous samples. If PCR is not available, Goldmann-Witmer coefficient may be calculated from intraocular antibody titers (6). If HIV status is unknown, HIV testing should be performed
- Treatment: Intravenous acyclovir or ganciclovir, with or without foscarnet, is commonly used but generally ineffective. Vitrectomy with

laser photocoagulation, with or without silicone oil or gas tamponade, may be considered for eyes with rhegmatogenous retinal detachment and visual potential

- Prognosis: Visual outcomes poor

CMV Retinitis

CMV retinitis, once a commonly observed opportunistic infection in end-stage AIDS patients, is now on the wane, thanks to the widespread use of highly active antiretroviral therapy (HAART). CMV retinitis occurs in AIDS and other patients with very low CD4$^+$ lymphocyte counts (usually less than 50/mm^3); however, is slow in progression and therefore has a better visual prognosis when compared with ARN and PORN. Nevertheless, visual outcomes may be limited

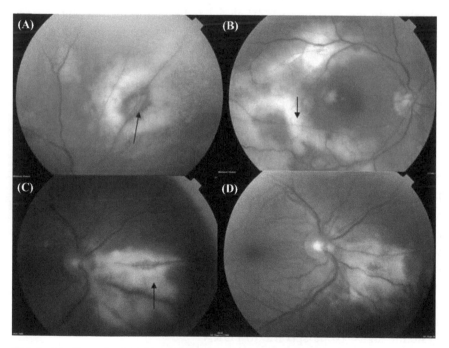

Figure 11 Fundal color photographic appearance of progressive outer retinal necrosis. (**A, B**) This post–bone marrow transplant patient presented with a herpetic retinal outer necrosis (*arrows*) with minimal vitritis that progressed with a retinal detachment requiring vitrectomy and silicon oil. A retinal biopsy and vitreous biopsy at the time confirmed infection with VZV and CMV herpes viruses. (**C, D**) PORN in a separate bone marrow transplant patient: lesions (*arrow*) resolved following systemic and intravitreal foscarnet therapy (**D**). *Abbreviations*: VZV, varicella-zoster virus; CMV, cytomegalovirus; PORN, progressive outer retinal necrosis.

by secondary retinal detachment. Some patients on immunosuppressive treatment, who develop CMV retinitis, may experience spontaneous regression of their retinitis with reduction or discontinuation of their immunosuppressive regimen. CMV retinitis may also develop in newborn infants with systemic CMV infection, which may be fatal, or may result in severe central nervous system sequelae. In general, there are two distinct presentations of active CMV retinitis. The first involves an edematous retinitis with anywhere from mild to prominent retinal hemorrhages, usually in one or two areas either starting in the periphery or in the peripapillary region. The second involves more indolent disease with a granular appearance to the retinitis and minimal retinal edema or hemorrhage. The latter may be difficult to distinguish from regressing disease and therefore requires careful evaluation. Frosted branch angiitis and immune recovery uveitis (IRU), both immune phenomena which can be observed in patients with CMV retinitis are described in separate sections. Finally, it should be noted that CMV retinitis in AIDS patients can occur concomitantly with other opportunistic retinal infections, mainly toxoplasmosis retinochoroiditis, cryptococcal retinitis, and HSV retinitis.

- Presenting symptoms: Decreased vision, peripheral scotoma
- Medical history/demographic associations: AIDS, immunosuppressive treatment for autoinflammatory disease, cancer treatment, newborn infants with systemic CMV infection
- Ocular signs: Bilateral in up to one-third of AIDS patients, although usually unilateral in patients on immunosuppressive therapy. *Anterior*: Minimal-to-no anterior segment inflammation. *Posterior*: Minimal-to-no vitritis, patchy retinal whitening and edema starting in the periphery or in the peripapillary area, commonly associated with retinal hemorrhages initially. Alternatively, a granular and somewhat faded pattern of retinitis starting in the periphery may be observed (Fig. 12). Without treatment, progressive enlargement and coalescence of lesions is observed over months. Vasculitis and papillitis are common features, particularly in later stages, with variable progression to vascular occlusion and optic atrophy
- Systemic signs: Fever, malaise, diarrhea, and abdominal pains (infective mononucleosis-like syndrome) may accompany acute systemic CMV infection
- Workup: PCR of aqueous or vitreous samples. If PCR is not available, Goldmann-Witmer coefficient may be calculated from intraocular antibody titers (6). If HIV status is unknown, HIV testing should be performed

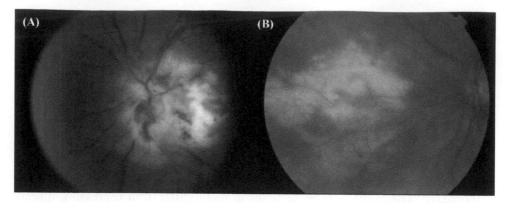

Figure 12 Fundal color photographs of CMV retinitis. (**A**) CMV retinitis affecting the optic nerve head. (**B**) Granular pattern of CMV retinitis in peripheral retina. *Abbreviation*: CMV, cytomegalovirus.

- Treatment: Intravenous gancyclovir induction followed by oral gancyclovir for maintenance. Intravitreal gancyclovir injection, intravitreal gancyclovir implant, oral valgancyclovir, intravenous or intravitreal foscarnet, and intravenous cidofovir are alternative therapies. Vitrectomy with laser photocoagulation, with or without silicone oil or gas tamponade, should be performed for rhegmatogenous retinal detachment in eyes with visual potential
- Prognosis: Varies depending on degree of posterior pole involvement and whether retinal detachment develops

Immune Recovery Uveitis

With the advent of the use of HAART in AIDS patients, a chronic vitritis termed IRU has been identified in AIDS patients with a history of treated, regressed CMV retinitis. A 19-center study of 274 patients with AIDS and CMV retinitis concluded that IRU occurred in roughly 17% of those patients who had immune recovery on HAART, defined as an increase of the CD4^{+} T-cell count by at least 50 cells/mm^3 to a level of at least 100 cells/mm^3 (9). Prior use of intravenous cidofovir appears to be a major risk factor for this disorder, although the reason for this association is unclear (9,10). More widespread CMV retinitis involvement also appears to be a predisposing factor, although anti-CMV treatment is not effective for IRU (9,10). PCR analysis of vitreous from these eyes has failed to identify CMV replication (11), supporting the current view that IRU is not recurrence of CMV infection but a noninfectious immune reaction in patients who have had reconstitution of immunity. IRU has been included here in the infectious disease section because of its close association with CMV retinitis. IRU responds well to local anti-inflammatory therapy without reactivation of CMV retinitis (12).

IRU has been reported in a non-AIDS immunosuppressed patient with previous CMV retinitis (13).

- Presenting symptoms: Decreased vision, floaters, photophobia
- Medical history/demographic associations: AIDS or immunosuppressed patient with immune reconstitution and treated, regressed CMV retinitis
- Ocular signs: Bilateral in roughly one-third of patients. *Anterior*: Minimal-to-moderate anterior segment inflammation. *Posterior*: Vitritis, cystoid macular edema, areas of healed CMV retinitis. Epiretinal membrane, proliferative vitreoretinopathy, retinal neovascularization, and vitreous hemorrhage may be observed in late stages
- Systemic signs: None specific to IRU.
- Workup: CD4$^+$ T-cell count. Consider aqueous or vitreous taps only if necessary to rule out active infection due to other organisms such as *Toxoplasma* or fungi
- Treatment: Topical and periocular injections of corticosteroids. Surgery should be performed for cataract, retinal detachment, and other complications
- Prognosis: Variable, depending on late complications

HIV Retinopathy

Systemic infection by the retrovirus HIV causes a mild, often asymptomatic, retinopathy in up to two-thirds of patients, which commonly resolves spontaneously (14). Deposition of circulating immune complexes, HIV infection of retinal vascular endothelial cells, and hemorheologic abnormalities have been suggested as possible pathogenic mechanisms for HIV retinopathy.

More than likely, the patient diagnosed with HIV retinopathy already has known HIV infection and is being referred to the ophthalmologist for screening. However, if HIV retinopathy is found in an individual with undiagnosed HIV infection, the patient should undergo a systemic workup for possible opportunistic infections and be assessed using the 1993 Revised Classification by the U.S. Centers for Disease Control (Table 2) (15). Category A consists of individuals with asymptomatic HIV infection, category B consists of patients with symptomatic HIV infection (such as fever or oral thrush) but no category C AIDS indicator conditions, and category C consists of patients with an AIDS indicator condition (such as *Pneumocystis* pneumonia and disseminated *Mycobacterium avium* complex infection). Category C patients and all patients regardless of category with a CD4$^+$ lymphocyte count of less than 200/mm^3 or 14% are classified as having AIDS. Newly diagnosed patients with HIV infection should also be screened for sexually transmitted diseases and receive counseling

Table 2 1993 Revised Classification for HIV Infection by the U.S. Centers for Disease Control

Category	General description	Representative symptoms/diseases
A	Asymptomatic HIV infection	None
B	Symptomatic HIV infection	Fever, diarrhea, oral candidiasis (thrush), oral hairy leukoplakia, cutaneous zoster, peripheral neuropathy
C	AIDS indicator condition	*Pneumocystis* pneumonia, toxoplasmic encephalitis, cryptococcal meningitis, disseminated *M. avium* complex infection, tuberculosis, recurrent bacterial pneumonia, disseminated cytomegalovirus infection, Burkitt's lymphoma, primary central nervous system lymphoma, invasive cervical carcinoma

Abbreviations: HIV, human immunodeficiency virus; AIDS, acquired immunodeficiency syndrome.
Source: From Ref. 15.

regarding sexual contact, the major mode of transmission today. Transmission may also occur via transfusion of blood products, sharing of needles by intravenous drug abusers, transplantation of infected grafts, and from mother to infant either intrauterine or peripartum.

HIV retinopathy must be distinguished from early infection due to toxoplasmosis, CMV, and other opportunistic organisms. While the cotton wool spots and retinal hemorrhages of HIV retinopathy spontaneously regress, with new lesions appearing perhaps months later, infections due to opportunistic organisms will progress in the absence of specific antimicrobial treatment.

- Presenting symptoms: A scotoma may be noted, but most often asymptomatic
- Medical history/demographic associations: Fever, diarrhea, weight loss, cutaneous zoster in a young individual or other evidence of opportunistic infections, intravenous drug abuser, sex industry worker, previous blood product transfusions, or transplantation procedures
- Ocular signs: Usually bilateral but may not occur simultaneously in both eyes. *Anterior*: No anterior segment inflammation. *Posterior*: Retinal hemorrhages, cotton wool spots
- Systemic signs: Fever, cough, thrush. HIV infection may be asymptomatic (category A)
- Workup: HIV antibody testing, complete blood count with white cell differential, $CD4^+$ lymphocyte count, syphilis and *Toxoplasma* serologies. Chest X ray and other tests should be considered based on symptoms and signs

- Treatment: No specific treatment necessary
- Prognosis: Visual outcomes good for HIV retinopathy

AIDS-Associated Ocular Conditions

Aside from HIV retinopathy described above, the following is a list of ocular conditions observed in HIV infection and AIDS patients. Please refer to the individual sections on specific diseases for descriptions.

- External: Dry eye, herpes zoster ophthalmicus, Kaposi's sarcoma of eyelid or conjunctiva, *Molluscum contagiosum*, periocular cutaneous zoster
- Intraocular: CMV retinitis, IRU, HSV or VZV retinitis, PORN, *Pneumocystis* choroiditis, cryptococcal choroiditis, toxoplasmosis, *M. avium-intracellulare* choroiditis, tuberculosis, syphilis, fungal infection, intraocular lymphoma

Human T Lymphocyte Virus Type 1 Uveitis

The human T lymphocyte virus type 1 (HTLV-1) is a retrovirus that causes a variety of diseases, most commonly adult T-cell leukemia/lymphoma (ATL) and HTLV-1-associated myopathy with onset usually in adulthood. HTLV-1 infection is also associated with inflammatory arthropathy, polymyositis, Graves' disease, Sjögren's syndrome, and a generalized increased susceptibility to infection. The virus may cause unilateral or bilateral intraocular inflammation manifesting predominantly as an indolent vitritis (intermediate uveitis) (16); since there is a high rate of asymptomatic seropositivity in endemic regions of the world, other known causes of intraocular inflammation must be ruled out first. HTLV-1 infection is endemic in southern Japan, southern New Zealand, northern Australia, West and Central Africa, the Caribbean basin, including southeastern United States, Mexico and northern South America, and the eastern part of South America. The primary modes of infection are sexual contact, transfusion of blood products, and breast-feeding, and familial clustering of disease is common. Of note, patients with ATL may develop CMV retinitis and intraocular lymphoma due to the progressive immunocompromised state.

- Presenting symptoms: Decreased vision, floaters
- Medical history/demographic associations: Resident of or parents from endemic area, sex industry worker, history of blood product transfusion
- Ocular signs: Bilateral in roughly one-half of patients. *Anterior*: Mild anterior segment inflammation. *Posterior*: Anterior or diffuse vitritis, retinal vasculitis, retinal sheathing, papillitis (Fig. 13), epiretinal membrane

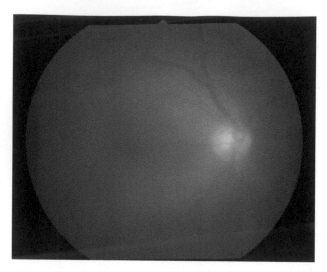

Figure 13 HTLV-1 uveitis. Mild vitritis (BIO 3), retinal vasculitis and papillitis are observed in this patient with HTLV-1-associated uveitis. *Abbreviation*: HTLV-1, human T lymphocyte virus type 1.

- Systemic signs: Lymphadenopathy and/or hepatosplenomegaly may suggest ATL
- Workup: Complete blood count including white cell differential, HTLV-1 antibody testing. Cerebrospinal fluid examination may reveal pleocytosis
- Treatment: Topical or periocular injections of corticosteroids are effective
- Prognosis: Generally good visual outcomes

Other Viral Diseases (Rubella, Subacute Sclerosing Panencephalitis, Measles, Mumps, Rift Valley Fever, Dengue Fever)

There are many other viruses that can cause PSII, although they are either rare or rarely observed outside specific endemic areas of the world.

- Congenital rubella (German measles) infection can cause a retinitis that is often only detected later as a quiescent salt-and-pepper appearance of the fundus, in a patient with normal or subnormal vision. Other ocular manifestations such as cataract and microphthalmos may be present.
- Subacute sclerosing panencephalitis, a progressive neurodegenerative disorder in primarily children caused by a variant of the measles virus can cause papillitis and retinal infiltrates.
- Acute acquired infection by either the measles or mumps virus can also manifest as a papillitis or neuroretinitis.

- The Rift Valley fever virus, borne by insects and endemic to eastern and southern Africa, can cause conjunctivitis and retinitis.
- The dengue fever virus is transmitted via mosquito bites in the endemic areas of Southeast Asia, Central and South America, and larger parts of coastal and southern Africa. Acute infection may be associated with retinal hemorrhages and papillitis (17).

Infectious Diseases: Bacterial

The overwhelming majority of bacterial infections causing predominantly PSII are chronic and indolent in nature. The important exception is endogenous bacterial endophthalmitis, which may progress quite rapidly. In the absence of a recent history of surgery or penetrating trauma to the eye (which is by far the commonest cause of bacterial endophthalmitis), a search for a systemic focus of metastatic infection (e.g., urinary bladder, bowel, gall bladder) is essential.

Bacterial Endophthalmitis

Bacterial endophthalmitis is usually a disease of acute onset presenting after intraocular surgery or penetrating eye injury (exogenous endophthalmitis), and is associated with predominantly anterior segment inflammation. Bacterial endophthalmitis that presents with predominantly PSII is most likely either delayed onset after cataract surgery (typically associated with *P. acnes* infection) or due to hematogenous spread from an infective source outside of the eye (endogenous or metastatic endophthalmitis). A slight majority of endogenous endophthalmitis is due to fungi (see sect. "Fungal Endophthalmitis") (18,19), while the remainder are due to bacteria, the most common being *Staphylococcus aureus*, *Streptococcus* species, and *Klebsiella* species. In the absence of ocular surgery or trauma, endogenous endophthalmitis should be suspected particularly in patients with a history of diabetes mellitus, valvular heart disease, recent hospitalization, nonocular surgery, and malignancies such as colon carcinoma. The following description pertains to endogenous bacterial endophthalmitis.

- Presenting symptoms: Ocular pain, red eye, floaters, decreased vision
- Medical history/demographic associations: Diabetes mellitus, meningitis, replaced heart valve, endocarditis, postoperative state (including after gastrointestinal endoscopy and dental procedures), intravenous hyper-alimentation, indwelling catheter, liver abscess, chronic renal failure, urinary tract infection, malignancy, intravenous drug abuse, alcoholism, newborn infants

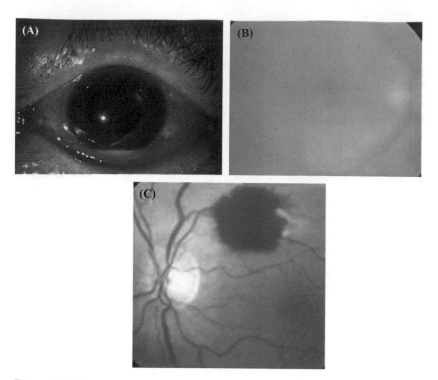

Figure 14 Color photographic composite of features of bacterial endophthalmitis. (**A**) Deeply red and painful inflamed eye with hypopyon. (**B**) Poor fundal view due to dense vitritis and (**C**) retinal hemorrhage in infiltrate in patient with culture positive bacterial endocarditis and endogenous endophthalmitis.

- Ocular signs: (Fig. 14) Bilateral in one-quarter of patients (20,21). *Anterior*: Eyelid swelling, conjunctival injection, chemosis, corneal edema, anterior chamber cells and fibrin with or without hypopyon, iris abscess, raised intraocular pressure, pupillary block glaucoma. *Posterior*: Focal or diffuse vitritis, retinal hemorrhages, retinal infiltrates, retinal necrosis, Roth spots. *Other*: Orbital involvement in severe cases
- Systemic signs: Fever and chills may be indicative of ongoing bacteremia
- Workup: Aqueous and/or vitreous stains and cultures, complete blood count with white cell differential. Stains and cultures of blood, urine, other bodily fluids (e.g., cerebrospinal fluid, ascites fluid), and implanted devices (e.g., central venous catheter), chest X ray and electrocardiogram should also be obtained as appropriate. In addition, cardiac ultrasonography (rule out valve abnormalities), abdominal ultrasonography

(rule out liver abscess, renal abnormalities, ascites, tumor), and gastro-intestinal endoscopy (rule out carcinoma) should be considered
- Common pathogens: *S. aureus*, *Streptococcus* species, *Klebsiella* species, *Neisseria meningitidis*, *Pseudomonas aeruginosa*, *Hemophilus influenzae*, *Escherichia coli*, *Bacillus cereus* (particular in intravenous drug users), *Nocardia asteroides* (patient on immunosuppression). The majority of organisms are gram-positive in North America and Europe while gram-negative in East Asia (22)
- Treatment: Specific antimicrobial therapy given topically, intravitreally, and/or intravenously based on clinical features and culture results. Intravenous therapy is generally needed for endogenous endophthalmitis. Vitrectomy may be considered in cases of severe vitreous opacification. Vitreous and other surgical specimens should be submitted for stains, culture, and/or pathological examination. Use of adjunctive cortico-steroids, either locally or systemically, may be considered
- Prognosis: Varies. Poor visual outcomes are associated with late detection (e.g., unconscious patient in intensive care unit) and certain virulent pathogens (e.g., *B. cereus*, *Serratia marcescens*, antibiotic-resistant *Staphylococcus*, and *Streptococcus* species)

Tuberculosis

Once believed to be the etiology of a majority of uveitis up through the first half of the 20th century, tuberculosis caused by the bacillus *M. tuberculosis* now accounts for a tiny fraction of diagnoses for ocular inflammation in the Western world. However, the fact that increasing antibiotic resistance is a serious problem particularly in AIDS patients, and the fact that tuberculosis is very much endemic in the vast majority of Asia, the Middle East, and Africa, tuberculosis should always remain in the differential diagnosis of any unexplained PSII. Still, intraocular inflammation is overall a very rare occurrence in tuberculosis and, in most cases, is believed to be due to an immune reaction to tuberculosis antigen elsewhere in the body. *M. tuberculosis* has been detected by PCR from a choroidal granuloma (23); however, in most cases isolation of the organism by ophthalmologists has been from eyelid or conjunctival lesions. Latent infection is common in endemic regions of the world, and difficulty in detecting and lack of a policy for treating such latent infection may be related to the continuing high prevalence of tuberculosis. Of note, Bacillus Calmette-Guerin (BCG) vaccination (usually given to children by health organizations at the national level) is only effective for the first 10 to 15 years (24) and makes interpretation of subsequent

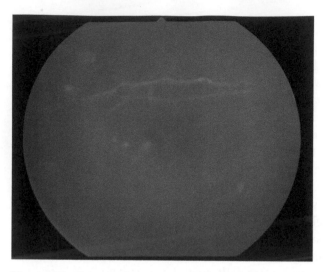

Figure 15 Color fundus photograph of tuberculosis associated vasculitis. Photograph represents old periphlebitis with "ghost vessel" formation in a patient with tuberculosis.

tuberculin purified protein derivative (PPD) skin testing difficult. A new test (Quantiferon®-TB Gold) involving assay of interferon-γ in whole blood incubated with a mixture of synthetic peptides representing two *M. tuberculosis* proteins appears to be useful in detecting latent infection (25). However, in the absence of positive results from such specific testing, pathological isolation, or PCR evidence of the bacillus from an ocular sample, the diagnosis remains "presumed" in most cases (26). Tuberculosis has been referred to as the "great masquerader" due to the variety of ocular manifestations with which it can present.

- Presenting symptoms: Red eye, ocular pain, decreased vision
- Medical history/demographic associations: Fever, night sweats, weight loss, malaise, productive cough, resident of or immigrant from an endemic region of the world
- Ocular signs: May be unilateral or bilateral. *Anterior*: Granulomatous anterior segment inflammation. *Posterior*: (Fig. 15; also see Fig. 3 of chap. 4) Diffuse vitritis, multifocal choroiditis, optic nerve granuloma, periphlebitis, retinal neovascularization, vitreous hemorrhage, diffuse choroiditis resembling serpiginous choroidopathy (often bilateral) (27). *Other*: Conjunctival or eyelid granuloma, nodular scleritis, keratitis
- Systemic signs: Fever in active systemic TB
- Workup: Complete blood count with white cell differential, erythrocyte sedimentation rate, C-reactive protein, PPD skin test, chest X ray or chest

computerized tomography, and sputum culture. Quantiferon®-TB Gold testing, if available, and PCR testing of ocular samples may be considered as appropriate

- Treatment: Current World Health Organization recommendations for persons not previously treated is two months of isoniazid, rifampicin, pyrazinamide, and ethambutol, followed by four months of isoniazid and rifampicin or isoniazid and ethambutol (28)
- Prognosis: Visual outcome varies depending on the ocular manifestations

Syphilis

Another disease of the old world that is still with us today is syphilis caused by the spirochete *Treponema pallidum*. With the advent of accurate diagnostic tests and penicillin therapy, this sexually transmitted disease has significantly waned in number, although remains a problem in certain segments of the population, particularly when found in AIDS patients in whom treatment beyond standard regimens may be required (29). Primary syphilis manifests as a genital or oral chancre accompanied by local lymphadenopathy, occurring roughly four weeks after primary infection. Secondary syphilis arises from hematogenous dissemination of the organism around 4 to 10 weeks after exposure, causing a generalized maculopapular or pustular rash, with varying degrees of fever, malaise, arthritis, and/or meningismus. Thereafter, the disease enters a latent phase, sometimes with recurrences of mucocutaneous lesions. Approximately 30% of patients with latent disease develop tertiary syphilis (late syphilis) with the development of gunmas (granulomatous skin lesions), cardiovascular lesions (aortitis, aortic aneurysm, valvular disease), and/or neurosyphilis (aseptic meningitis, cranial nerve palsies, Argyll Robertson pupil, encephalitis, tabes dorsalis). Congenital syphilis occurs with transplacental transmission to the fetus of *T. pallidum* from a mother with untreated primary or secondary syphilis, and manifests most commonly in the eye as salt-and-pepper chorioretinitis or bilateral interstitial keratitis in the newborn infant. Although said to be pathognomonic of congenital syphilis, Hutchinson's triad consisting of Hutchinson's teeth, interstitial keratitis, and deafness is rare. Like tuberculosis, syphilis can present with a wide variety of manifestations, mimicking many diseases. Ocular manifestations occur mostly in the secondary and tertiary phases of syphilis.

- Presenting symptoms: Decreased vision, unseeing newborn infant
- Medical history/demographic associations: Sex industry workers, AIDS, child abuse
- Ocular signs: Roughly one-half of PSII due to syphilis is bilateral. *Anterior*: Iridocyclitis, iris nodules. *Posterior*: Salt-and-pepper chorioretinitis, vitritis,

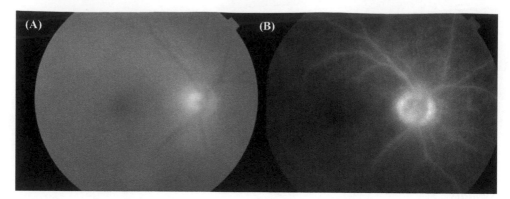

Figure 16 Color and flourescein angiogram fundal signs in syphilis. (**A**) Active retinal vasculitis involving mainly the veins, accompanied by papillitis and mild vitritis, in a patient with newly diagnosed syphilis. (**B**) Fluorescein angiogram showing prominent vascular and disc leakage. (With permission, Folia Ophthalmologica Japanica, Osaka)

peripapillary neuroretinitis, vasculitis (Fig. 16), retinal vascular occlusions, necrotizing retinitis, serous retinal detachment. *Other*: Eyelid or conjunctival chancre (rare presentation in primary syphilis only), blepharitis, conjunctivitis, scleritis, bilateral interstitial keratitis with ghost vessels (congenital syphilis), Argyll Robertson pupil

- Systemic signs: Mucocutaneous lesions, congenital neurological abnormalities in a newborn infant
- Workup: The Venereal Disease Research Laboratory (VDRL) test and rapid plasma reagin (RPR) test (nontreponemal tests) are used to detect anticardiolipin antibodies elicited in response to membrane lipids of *T. pallidum*. The fluorescein treponemal antibody absorption (FTA-ABS) test and the microhemagglutination–*T. pallidum* (MHA-TP) test (treponemal tests) are specific for detecting anti–*T. pallidum* antibodies. The VDRL and RPR tests may be false-positive in many situations, including pregnancy, other spirochetal infections, and mononucleosis, and will usually turn negative after treatment. The FTA-ABS and MHA-TP tests are much more sensitive especially for latent or tertiary syphilis, but may also be false-positive in patients with diseases such as rheumatoid arthritis, systemic lupus erythematosus, and biliary cirrhosis. The VDRL test may be performed on cerebrospinal fluid to rule out neurosyphilis. Patients (and their partners) suspected of sexual transmission should also be assessed for possible HIV, HSV, chlamydia, and gonorrhea infections
- Treatment: Oral (primary or secondary) or intravenous (tertiary syphilis) penicillin
- Prognosis: Visual outcomes generally good unless optic atrophy ensues

Lyme Disease

Lyme disease is a systemic infection caused by the spirochete *Borrelia burgdorferi*, which is borne by *Ixodes* ticks endemic to deer and many other wildlife populations, originally found in the northeastern United States but now recognized to be in many areas of the world. The initial tick bite is usually manifest by the skin lesion erythema migrans, which can last for three to four weeks (stage 1). This may be followed by hematogenous dissemination of the spirochetes, causing neurological symptoms (commonly headache and meningismus) and rarely cardiac abnormalities (such as heart block) within days to weeks (stage 2). A chronic arthritis phase may then ensue (stage 3), leading to further neurological symptoms and general chronic fatigue. Ocular abnormalities can occur at any stage of the disease, but most commonly involves conjunctivitis presenting in the early phase of disease (stages 1–2). Intraocular inflammation, with vitritis as the predominant feature in most cases, occurs in the late phase of disease (stage 3) (30,31).

- Presenting symptoms: Red eye, photophobia, periocular pain, floaters, decreased vision, diplopia
- Medical history/demographic associations: Recent tick bite, recent visit to or living in an endemic area
- Ocular signs: The intraocular inflammation due to Lyme disease is usually bilateral. *Anterior*: Conjunctivitis, episcleritis, iridocyclitis, keratitis. *Posterior*: Anterior or diffuse vitritis, retinal vasculitis, optic neuritis, choroiditis. *Other*: Bell's palsy (cranial nerve VII palsy), ocular motility disorders (due to cranial nerve III, IV, or VI palsy), orbital inflammation, cortical blindness
- Systemic signs: Skin lesion consistent with tick bite (erythema migrans), headache, stiff neck, arthralgias, chronic fatigue especially in association with neurological abnormalities
- Workup: Enzyme-linked immunosorbent assay (ELISA) for *B. burgdorferi* IgM and IgG antibodies. False-positive results may occur due to cross-reactions between *B. burgdorferi* and other spirochetes such as *T. pallidum*, so the FTA-ABS should also be checked to rule out syphilis
- Treatment: Topical, periocular and/or systemic corticosteroids for intraocular inflammation. For refractory inflammation, particularly in the early phase of disease, a course of systemic antibiotics (usually a macrolide or amoxicillin given orally) should be considered if the patient has never undergone specific treatment for Lyme disease. Neurological and cardiac disease may require intravenous antibiotics (penicillin or ceftriaxone). After a known tick bite, doxycycline prophylaxis may be considered
- Prognosis: Ocular inflammation is usually controllable using local corticosteroid therapy, with a generally favorable visual prognosis

Bartonella henselae

Cat scratch disease (a regional lymphadenopathy with flu-like symptoms) and the associated neuroretinitis, which can develop days to weeks later, were recognized in the early 1990s to be caused by the gram-negative bacillus *B. henselae*. *B. henselae* infection is endemic to not only cats (and kittens), but also cat fleas, dogs, monkeys, porcupines, and other wildlife (32). Ocular disease occurs in a small fraction of cat scratch disease patients and can manifest as conjunctivitis during the acute lymphadenopathy phase of disease. A distinctive papillitis followed by a macular star configuration of hard exudates may be observed later in the disease course. Papillitis with peripapillary serous retinal detachment (and no macular star) may predominate in the early phase of disease.

- Presenting symptoms: Decreased vision, photophobia, flashing lights, floaters
- Medical history/demographic associations: Fever, malaise, other flu-like symptoms, cat scratch, or other animal exposure
- Ocular signs: The neuroretinitis observed in *B. henselae* infection may be unilateral or bilateral. *Anterior*: Usually no anterior segment inflammation. *Posterior*: Retinal or choroidal white lesions, papillitis, macular star (Fig. 17), mild peripapillary serous retinal detachment, mild vitritis,

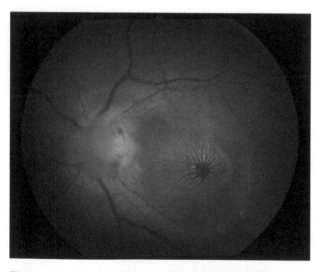

Figure 17 Neuroretinitis secondary to *Bartonella henselae*. An inflamed optic disc and macular star were observed in this patient one month after the onset of fever and flu-like symptoms. Antibiotic therapy was initiated and positive serum titers for *B. henselae* IgM and IgG later confirmed the diagnosis of cat scratch disease.

retinal vascular occlusion, choroidal granuloma (rare). *Other*: Conjunctival granuloma (acute lymphadenopathy phase)

- Systemic signs: Fever, lymphadenopathy
- Workup: Antibody or PCR testing for *B. henselae* and *Bartonella quintana* (the latter is useful as a control and is the etiology of related diseases such as bacillary angiomatosis)
- Treatment: Oral doxycycline, erythromycin, ciprofloxacin, rifampicin, and trimethoprim-sulfamethoxazole have all been used successfully, often in combination. Oral corticosteroids may be considered in selected cases
- Prognosis: Visual outcomes generally good

Other Bacteria (Tropheryma whippelii, N. asteroides, Brucella species, Rickettsia rickettsii)

Other much rarer bacterial infections that can cause predominantly PSII include the following:

- The gram-negative bacteria *T. whippelii* is the cause of Whipple's disease (or intestinal lipodystrophy), which manifests as chronic diarrhea, abdominal pain, and weight loss mostly in middle-aged men. Ocular manifestations include vitritis, retinitis, and multifocal choroiditis. Central nervous system involvement causing cranial nerve palsies, nystagmus, and optic neuritis may also occur.
- Brucellosis is caused by the gram-negative bacteria *Brucella melitensis* or *Brucella abortis* and is a zoonotic disease transferred to humans through unpasteurized milk or raw meat. A systemic flu-like illness develops followed by anterior segment inflammation and multifocal choroiditis.
- *N. asteroides* is a gram-positive bacteria that can cause disseminated infection in immunocompromised hosts such as patients with malignancies and AIDS. Ocular manifestations include anterior segment inflammation, vitritis, chorioretinitis, and choroidal abscesses.
- The bacteria *R. rickettsii* borne by ticks in both North and South America is the etiological agent of Rocky Mountain spotted fever. Ocular manifestations include conjunctivitis, anterior segment inflammation, retinal hemorrhages, retinal cotton wool spots, and papillitis.

Infectious Diseases: Fungal

As with many bacterial infections affecting the posterior eye, fungal diseases tend to be of slow onset, and some cases may be asymptomatic.

Fungal Endophthalmitis

Fungi represent the etiological agent for a slight majority of cases of infectious endogenous endophthalmitis (18,19). Fungal endophthalmitis generally occurs in a patient with obvious predisposing medical history, such as recent major surgery, intravenous hyperalimentation, or indwelling catheter. Some of these patients may be unconscious or otherwise unaware of ocular symptoms, leading to late detection. However, the infection is slowly progressive in nature and amenable to appropriate antimicrobial therapy with adjunctive surgery when necessary.

- Presenting symptoms: Decreased vision, floaters
- Medical history/demographic associations: Diabetes mellitus, intravenous hyperalimentation, indwelling catheter, postoperative state (especially after gastrointestinal surgery), chronic renal failure, chronic pulmonary disease, intravenous drug abuse, cancer or immunosuppression treatment, neonate, postpartum women, prolonged antibiotic use
- Ocular signs: Bilateral in two-thirds of patients. *Anterior*: Usually mild to no anterior segment inflammation. *Posterior*: Any type of vitritis, large "fungus balls" in the vitreous, retinal infiltrates (Fig. 18), vitreoretinal adhesions, papillitis, multifocal choroiditis (*Cryptococcus neoformans*)
- Systemic signs: Chronic systemic disease, fever
- Workup: Vitreous sampling for stains and cultures, complete blood count with white cell differential. Serum *Candida* antigen and β-D-glucan (33) testing may be useful to identify ongoing candidemia. Stains and cultures of blood, urine, other bodily fluids (e.g., ascites fluid) and implanted devices (e.g., central venous catheter) should be performed as appropriate

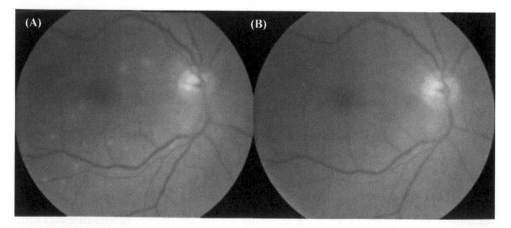

Figure 18 Fundal color photographs showing successful resolution of fungal endophthalmitis. Multifocal retinal infiltrates in a patient who had been on intravenous hyperalimentation. (**A**) Initial presentation. (**B**) After treatment with oral fluconazole.

- Common pathogens: Three-quarters due to *Candida* species (*Candida albicans* or *Candida parapsilosis*). Other fungi include *Aspergillus fumigatus*, *Blastomyces dermatitidis*, *Coccidioides immitis*, *Sporothrix schenckii*, and *C. neoformans*
- Treatment: Intravenous amphotericin B, or oral fluconazole, flucytosine, or voraconazole. Vitrectomy and intravitreal amphotericin B administration may be considered in cases with dense vitritis
- Prognosis: Good visual outcomes in eyes with timely detection and treatment, and absence of foveal lesions

Ocular Histoplasmosis and Histoplasmosis-Like Disease

Ocular histoplasmosis is a diagnosis based purely on characteristic clinical features and circumstantial evidence in that these patients have been found to have a high rate of antibodies or positive skin test results indicative of exposure to *Histoplasma capsulatum*, a fungus transmitted to humans by air-borne spores and endemic to the Ohio–Mississippi River valleys of the United States. However, in all likelihood, a similar pattern of disease can be caused by a variety of fungal organisms. For example, similar fundus findings have been documented in European patients living in areas that are not endemic for *H. capsulatum* (34), and these cases have been classified as histoplasmosis-like disease until the causative organism is found. In either situation, the majority of patients are identified either incidentally with inactive scars only or presenting with visual loss due to secondary choroidal neovascularization (CNV) in the macula. Rarely, a patient with typical features may have choroidal lesions that show active inflammation.

- Presenting symptoms: Often asymptomatic, decreased vision with foveal lesion
- Medical history/demographic associations: Healthy individual, may be current or prior resident of Ohio–Mississippi regions
- Ocular signs: Usually bilateral, but involvement may be asymmetric. *Anterior*: No anterior segment inflammation. *Posterior*: Absence of vitreous cells, punched-out atrophic chorioretinal lesions ("histo spots"), linear chorioretinal scars at the equator, peripapillary atrophy, CNV usually involving the fovea. All types of lesions have prominent pigmentation
- Systemic signs: None
- Workup: Fluorescein angiography for suspicion of CNV
- Treatment: Photodynamic therapy (35), intravitreal/periocular injections of corticosteroids (36), or systemic immunosuppression (37) may be considered for CNV. Intravitreal injection of anti–vascular endothelial

growth factor (VEGF) agents such as ranibizumab or bevacizumab may also be effective, although specific data in eyes with ocular histoplasmosis is lacking
- Prognosis: Visual outcomes good unless CNV develops

Pneumocystis

Once believed to be a protozoan, sequence analysis of various proteins has shown that *Pneumocystis* is more closely related to fungi, although with important distinctions from traditional fungi that make *Pneumocystis* resistant to many antifungal agents. *Pneumocystis* pneumonia is a common opportunistic infection in AIDS patients, previously thought to be caused by *Pneumocystis carinii* but now known to be due to *Pneumocystis jiroveci* (38). Extrapulmonary spread can occur to other organs including the eyes where it may cause multifocal infectious foci in the choroid (39) that slowly enlarge and coalesce if left untreated. *Pneumocystis* choroiditis may be encountered in AIDS patients whose *Pneumocystis* pneumonia prophylaxis consists only of aerosolized pentamidine and not oral trimethoprim-sulfamethoxazole (40). Fortunately, the disease responds well to systemic administration of appropriate antibiotics, although is indicative of a state of severe immunosuppression in the patient.

- Presenting symptoms: Decreased vision or mild blurring, may be asymptomatic
- Medical history/demographic associations: AIDS or immunocompromised state
- Ocular signs: Unilateral or bilateral. *Anterior*: None. *Posterior*: No vitritis, usually multiple yellow-white subretinal plaques in the posterior pole, occasionally serous retinal detachment. *Other*: May occur concurrently with CMV retinitis in the same or fellow eye
- Systemic signs: Fever and malaise indicative of disseminated fungal infection
- Workup: Evaluation for *Pneumocystis* infection in other organs
- Treatment: Intravenous trimethoprim-sulfamethoxazole or intravenous pentamidine
- Prognosis: Visual outcomes may be good

Infectious Diseases: Parasitic

Human parasitic infections are zoonotic diseases, i.e., occur via transmission of the offending organism from a reservoir in animals. The diseases in this category occur mainly in populations with close contact to infected animals (children playing with infected pets or in sandboxes soiled by infected feces) or in areas of the world where the consumption of raw meat (Europe, East Asia) or the household preparation of meat sausages (South America) are common.

Toxoplasmosis

Despite a high rate of seropositivity to *Toxoplasma gondii*, this protozoan causes symptomatic disease in only 10% to 20% of infected individuals (41). The rate and severity of disease increases dramatically with AIDS and other immunocompromised states, such as malignancy, and can unfortunately cause major congenital abnormalities (including intracranial calcifications, hydrocephalus, bilateral macular scars) in infants born to mothers with new and untreated infection particularly when acquired during the first or second trimesters (congenital toxoplasmosis). However, the vast majority of infections are acquired, asymptomatic, and occur in immunocompetent adults, resulting in latent infection that may reactivate. Three forms of the organism exist: the oocyst that releases sporozoites, the tissue cyst that contains and may release bradyzoites, and the tachyzoite. Transmission to humans commonly occurs from the cat in which the sexual cycle of *T. gondii* occurs. Oocytes released into cat feces infect the gastrointestinal tract of humans directly via ingestion of contaminated soil or indirectly through consumed raw or undercooked meats, particularly pork. *T. gondii* is also found in chicken, goats, deer, bears, and most other wildlife, and transmission to humans by transport hosts such as cockroaches and flies is also suspected. Consumption of raw vegetables contaminated by oocysts may also occur. Toxoplasmosis accounts for more than 85% of all patients with posterior uveitis in southern Brazil (42) and is also particularly common in France. Pregnant women and immunosuppressed patients should undergo systematic screening for *T. gondii*.

- Presenting symptoms: Decreased vision, floaters, photophobia
- Medical history/demographic associations: Rarely a history of fever, malaise, night sweats. Farm or meat industry workers, AIDS, malignancy, organ transplantation, small children, newborn infants, residents of *T. gondii* endemic area
- Ocular signs: Acute reactivation is usually unilateral although old scars may be found in both eyes (Fig. 19). *Anterior*: Mild-to-moderate granulomatous anterior segment inflammation. *Posterior*: Mild-to-severe focal or diffuse vitritis (Fig. 2; also see Fig. 2 of chap. 4), solitary whitish retinal infiltrate usually near a pigmented atrophic scar, retinal vasculitis, papillitis. May rarely present as an ARN (4). CNV associated with a quiescent macular scar may occur but is uncommon

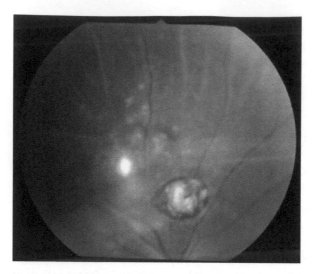

Figure 19 Fundus color photograph of *Toxoplasma* chorioretinitis. Reactivation of toxoplasmosis. Note the new white retinal infiltrates near an old chorioretinal scar. (With permission, Igaku-Shoin Medical Publishers, Tokyo)

- Systemic signs: Occasionally lymphadenopathy and hepatosplenomegaly in acute primary infection, but usually no systemic symptoms in immunocompetent individuals. Neurological abnormalities may be evident in AIDS or immunosuppressed patients with CNS involvement
- Workup: Serum antibodies to *T. gondii*. Elevated IgM titers would indicate new infection, while elevated IgG titers would only suggest reactivation. PCR of intraocular fluids may be performed for atypical presentations. Brain MRI should be considered in AIDS and other immunocompromised patients to rule out toxoplasmic intracranial abscesses
- Treatment: Common treatment regimens include (*i*) "triple therapy" involving pyrimethamine (with folinic acid to counter the adverse effect of bone marrow suppression), sulfadiazine and prednisolone depending on the degree of active inflammation, (*ii*) triple therapy plus clindamycin, (*iii*) substitution of the sulfadiazine in triple therapy with clindamycin, clarithromycin, atovaquone, azithromycin, or dapsone, (*iv*) trimethoprim-sulfamethoxazole, and (*v*) spiramycin, which is the drug of choice in pregnancy. Although the chorioretinal reactivation itself is self-limiting, all acute recurrences should be treated in order to limit tissue damage and to theoretically inhibit the formation of new retinal tissue cysts. Prophylaxis using trimethoprim-sulfamethoxazole (43) should be considered in AIDS and other immunocompromised patients, and in pregnant women who show serological conversion with a positive IgM titer.

Long-term intermittent trimethoprim-sulfamethoxazole treatment may also be useful in patients with recurrent disease (44)

- Prognosis: Poor visual outcomes for foveal involvement and immuno-compromised patients

Toxocariasis

Toxocariasis is a helminthic infection caused by the roundworm *Toxocara canis*, which is endemic to dogs and related animals such as foxes and wolves. Transmission to humans occurs via the ingestion of eggs found in feces or vomitus of infected animals, particularly puppies that are known to actively shed eggs. Toxocariasis may occur with close contact to infected animals, ingestion of contaminated soil, contaminated hands or utensils, or ingestion of uncooked food. In both animals and humans, the eggs hatch in the small intestines, with subsequent hematological and lymphatic migration of resulting larva to the liver, lungs, trachea, lymph nodes, and eyes. Humans do not harbor adult worms or excrete eggs. The majority of individuals acutely infected with *T. canis* are asymptomatic or only have mild flu-like symptoms. However, the infection can be symptomatic with the onset of visceral larva migrans (VLM), a disorder characterized by fever, lymphadenopathy, hepatosplenomegaly, and eosinophilia, usually found in small children under the age of six years. Ocular symptoms are rare in acute VLM. More commonly, ocular toxocariasis is found in otherwise healthy children being worked up for leukocoria in the absence of a history of VLM (45).

- Presenting symptoms: Leukocoria, strabismus, decreased vision
- Medical history/demographic associations: Young children, exposure to dogs and cats, playground exposure
- Ocular signs (Fig. 20): Usually unilateral. *Anterior*: Mild-to-no anterior segment inflammation. *Posterior*: Mild-to-no vitritis, posterior pole or peripheral whitish inflammatory mass (granuloma), with or without vitreoretinal traction extending to the disc, tractional retinal detachment, epiretinal membrane, cyclitic membrane with hypotony. Occasionally, a severe diffuse vitritis (endophthalmitis) can occur, and rarely a granuloma can be centered on the optic disc. *Other*: Strabismus
- Systemic signs: None
- Workup: Serological testing for antibodies to *T. canis*. If cataract is present, B scan ultrasonography may aid in the workup of leukocoria since intraocular calcification is not observed in ocular toxocariasis but is a feature in retinoblastoma
- Treatment: Systemic or periocular injections of corticosteroids may be considered for severe vitritis. Specific antihelminthic therapy is generally

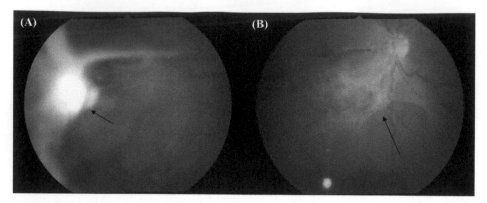

Figure 20 Fundal color photographs presenting appearance following *Toxocara* infection. (**A**) Peripheral granuloma formation (*arrow*) and (**B**) extensive epiretinal membrane formation (*arrow*) in an eye with a peripheral *Toxocara* granuloma. (With permission, Igaku-Shoin Medical Publishers, Tokyo)

ineffective. Surgery may be considered for secondary cataract, severe vitritis, and/or tractional retinal detachment

- Prognosis: Variable, poor visual outcomes for foveal lesions, traction retinal detachment, dragged macula, and hypotony

Other Parasitic Diseases (Diffuse Unilateral Subacute Neuroretinitis, Onchocerciasis, Cysticercosis, Ophthalmomyiasis, Echinococcosis, Amebiasis)

There are numerous other parasites that can directly infect the ocular tissues, most occurring in residents of or travelers to tropical regions of the world. Onchocerciasis in particular is a major cause of impaired vision or blindness in the developing world.

- Diffuse unilateral subacute neuroretinitis is a disorder caused by the nematode *Baylisascaris procyonis* and other helminths as well, most commonly diagnosed in the southeastern United States and the Caribbean. The disease manifests as yellow-white outer retinal infiltrates with retinal vasculitis and papillitis in the acute phase. A diffuse pigmented RPE degeneration with optic atrophy or geographic pigmented subretinal fibrosis is observed in the late phase.
- Onchocerciasis, also called "river blindness," is caused by the filarial nematode *Onchocerca volvulus. O. volvulus* is transmitted by the biting blackfly that breeds around rivers and streams and is endemic in much of Africa, the eastern Mediterranean, and Central and South America. The disease manifests as a maculopapular rash that leads to a distinctive

pigmentary change of the skin over years, subcutaneous nodules, lymphadenopathy, and corneal and intraocular infiltration of microfilariae with end-stage pigmented chorioretinal atrophy.

- Cysticercosis is caused by the encystment of the larva *Cysticercus cellulosae* from the tapeworm *Taenia solium*, mainly transmitted by ingesting eggs in food or water contaminated by human feces. Disseminated larva form cysts in muscle, the central nervous system, and the eyes where intraocular cysts can be observed in the vitreous or subretinal space.

- Ophthalmomyiasis is caused by infiltration of the ocular (ophthalmomyiasis interna) or periocular (ophthalmomyiasis externa) tissues by the larva (maggots) of many different fly species that are deposited in the skin of animals such as sheep or rotting organic materials, and occurs in roughly 5% of cases of myasis or systemic maggot infection. Manifestations include conjunctivitis, keratitis, a criss-crossing pattern of retinopathy, tractional retinal detachment, and orbital infection depending on the larva type.

- Echinococcosis is caused by ingestion of eggs of the *Echinococcus* species, which are cestodes carried by tapeworms endemic to dogs and other canines. The eggs hatch oncospheres that penetrate the intestinal mucosa and encyst in liver, lung, and other organs, including the eye with accompanying chorioretinitis.

- Amebiasis is caused by *Entamoeba histolytica* (different from the organism *Acanthomoeba* that causes contact lens wear–associated keratitis), and can in rare instances cause a choroiditis with secondary vitritis and papillitis.

Presumed Autoinflammatory Diseases, with Systemic Manifestations

Presumed autoinflammatory diseases form an ill-defined category that encompasses disorders presumed to be either primary dysfunctions of immunity or dysfunctions secondary to infectious or other environmental triggers. Many of these diseases have human leukocyte antigen (HLA) associations, and therefore are common to specific ethnic groups and/or regions of the world. In particular, presumed autoinflammatory diseases account for a majority of PSII (posterior uveitis or panuveitis) in large surveys published from countries such as Japan and Italy (46,47). Diseases that are primarily systemic disorders or that have significant systemic manifestations are described in this section. Note that all of these diseases are overwhelmingly bilateral, although both eyes may not be affected with active intraocular inflammation at the same time.

Behçet's Disease

Behçet's disease is a chronic multisystem disease consisting of recurrent oral ulcers (aphthae), recurrent genital ulcers, a variety of skin disorders, and chronic/recurrent anterior and posterior intraocular inflammation. It is most commonly diagnosed in countries that line the Old Silk Road stretching from the Mediterranean through the Middle East to Eastern Asia. There appears to be some genetic susceptibility as the disease is associated with the HLA-B51 haplotype, although the strength of this association depends on the population being examined. However, exogenous factors, particularly infections are also suspected of contributing to the pathogenesis of disease. Clinical onset of disease usually occurs in the third to fourth decades of life, with men being more commonly afflicted than women. The ocular disease is believed to be particularly severe in young adult men and, although the disease may start out unilaterally, it eventually manifests with bilateral intraocular inflammation in most patients. Behçet's disease can be particularly debilitating when the central nervous system becomes involved, and it can also cause arthritis, gastrointestinal ulcers, systemic large vessel occlusion, vascular aneurysms, epididymitis, and myocarditis. Behçet's disease is diagnosed based on clinical features alone, as there are no specific ancillary tests. An international collaborative published one set of diagnostic criteria that are commonly used (Table 3) (48).

- Presenting symptoms: Decreased vision, floaters, photophobia
- Medical history/demographic associations: Recurrent painful mouth or genital ulcers, fever, skin disorders. Mediterranean, Middle Eastern, or Asian heritage
- Ocular signs (Fig. 21): Bilateral in approximately 90% of patients, but with recurrences occurring in one eye at a time. *Anterior*: Recurrent anterior segment nongranulomatous inflammation, with or without hypopyon. Posterior iris synechia may be observed. *Posterior*: Diffuse vitritis, retinal vasculitis, retinal infiltrates (Fig. 5), retinal hemorrhages, and/or papillitis with acute attacks. Retinal vascular sheathing and/or occlusion, retinal neovascularization, epiretinal membrane, optic and macular atrophy in late stages (Fig. 21). Retinal vascular occlusion can lead to peripheral areas of nonperfusion and retinal neovascularization. *Other*: Ocular motility dysfunction or ptosis may occasionally occur due to cranial nerve palsy
- Systemic signs: Fever, malaise, oral ulcers, genital ulcers, erythema nodosum, subcutaneous thrombophlebitis, acneiform lesions
- Workup: Fluorescein angiography often shows diffuse capillary leakage even in the absence of an acute attack. HLA-B51 testing may be considered with appropriate consultations for specific systemic manifestations

Table 3 International Study Group Criteria for the Diagnosis of Behçet's Disease (48)

Finding[a]	Definition
Recurrent oral ulceration	Minor aphthous, major aphthous, or herpetiform ulcers observed by the physician or patient, which have recurred at least 3 times over a 12-month period
Plus at least two of the following criteria:	
Recurrent genital ulceration	Aphthous ulceration or scarring observed by physician or patient
Eye lesions	Anterior uveitis, posterior uveitis or cells in vitreous on slit lamp examination; or retinal vasculitis detected by an ophthalmologist
Skin lesions	Erythema nodosum observed by physician or patient, pseudofolliculitis, or papulopustular lesions; or acneiform nodules observed by physician in postadolescent patients not on corticosteroid treatment
Positive pathergy test[b]	Interpreted by the physician at 24 to 48 hr

[a]Findings applicable only in absence of other clinical explanations.
[b]Also referred to as the "skin prick" or "Behçetine" test and involves a nonspecific inflammatory reaction to a needle prick or an intradermal injection of saline.

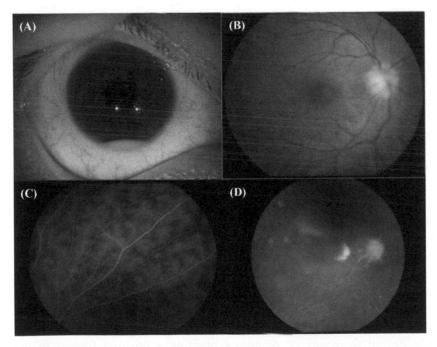

Figure 21 Composite of ocular features of Behçet's disease. (**A**) Painless hypopyon during an acute anterior segment attack. (**B**) Acute papillitis. (**C**) Diffuse capillary dye leakage on fluorescein angiography as shown here is typically observed in eyes with Behçet's disease, even during periods without clinically observable intraocular inflammation. (**D**) Optic atrophy and severe vascular fibrosis.

- Treatment: Acute inflammatory attacks are generally self-limiting. However, attacks of the posterior segment, particularly when involving areas in the macula or involving the optic disc, should be aggressively treated with sub-Tenon's or intravitreal corticosteroid administration in order to limit permanent damage to central visual function. Furthermore, in patients with posterior attacks, systemic therapy using cyclosporine or other immunosuppressive agents (49), with or without low-dose corticosteroids, interferon-α (50), or tumor necrosis factor-α inhibition with infliximab (51) should be instituted early to improve the long-term visual outcome. Retinal neovascularization may regress with scatter laser photocoagulation to areas of nonperfusion, if present (52)
- Prognosis: Visual outcomes vary, but appear to be worst in young adult men. However, early and aggressive treatment with interferon-α (50) or infliximab (51) have shown excellent results (see chap. 5)

Sarcoidosis

Sarcoidosis is a chronic multisystem disease that presents with noncaseating granuloma formation most commonly in the lungs, thoracic lymph nodes, skin, and eyes, but may occur in virtually any organ system in the body. Particularly severe consequences can develop when the cardiac or central nervous system is involved. Ocular features may be the sole identifiable manifestation of the disease, and may be present in up to two-thirds of sarcoidosis patients. The disease is common in individuals of African, Hispanic, and Asian descent, and affects more women than men. Most patients present in adulthood, although sarcoidosis can occur in children and be misdiagnosed as juvenile rheumatoid arthritis. Although the etiology of disease is unknown, research has suggested that various microorganisms such as *M. tuberculosis* (53) and *P. acnes* (54) may trigger an immune response, leading to disease. Intraocular inflammation may be mild and asymptomatic in many patients, although in severe cases can cause permanent visual loss particularly due to glaucoma, either due to the disease itself or as a side effect of local corticosteroid therapy. Although elevation of serum angiotensin-converting enzyme (ACE) levels support a diagnosis of sarcoidosis, the ACE can be elevated in a variety of diseases, including tuberculosis, silicosis, primary biliary cirrhosis, hyperthyroidism, and liver cirrhosis. There are no international diagnostic criteria for the diagnosis of ocular sarcoidosis at present, and the only definitive means of diagnosis remains a positive biopsy in the absence of other causes of granulomatous disease. There is a hereditary sarcoidosis-like disease, known as familial juvenile systemic granulomatosus or

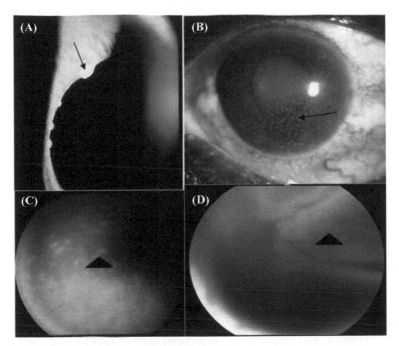

Figure 22 Composite color photographs demonstrating features of ocular sarcoidosis. (**A**) Multiple iris (Koeppe) nodules (*arrow*). (**B**) Conjunctival injection and mutton fat keratic precipitates (*arrow*) in a patient with sarcoidosis who presents with chronic bilateral anterior uveitis. (**C**) Typical chorioretinal exudates and vasculitis in the inferior retina. (**D**) Exudative retinal detachment. This is a rare ocular manifestation of sarcoidosis.

Blau syndrome, causing polyarthritis, panuveitis, skin rash, and camptodactyly presenting in childhood (55).

- Presenting symptoms: Redness, floaters, photophobia, decreased vision, lid droop, double vision; ocular disease may be asymptomatic
- Medical history/demographic associations: African, Hispanic, or Asian descent
- Ocular signs (Fig. 22): Almost always bilateral. *Anterior*: Granulomatous anterior segment inflammation, with keratic precipitates, iris nodules, peripheral anterior synechia, and/or posterior synechia being quite prominent in some cases. *Posterior*: Anterior or diffuse vitritis often with "snowballs" inferiorly (Fig. 2B), pars plana exudation, perivasculitis, retinal hemorrhages, choroidal infiltrates, particularly in the inferior periphery, solitary choroidal or disc granuloma (Fig. 3), epiretinal membrane, retinal detachment whether tractional, exudative, or rhegmatogenous. Of note, the perivasculitis in sarcoidosis tends to be

nonocclusive, in contrast to that seen in Behçet's disease or tuberculosis, and therefore is less associated with visual loss due to neovascularization or ischemia. *Other*: Lacrimal gland swelling, orbital inflammation, nasolacrimal duct obstruction, ptosis or ocular motility disorders (due to cranial nerve palsy), lid or conjunctival nodules

- Systemic signs: Fever, malaise, and dyspnea may be present, although most patients appear healthy. Subcutaneous nodules or erythema nodosum may be observed, particularly on the extremities
- Workup: Serum ACE, calcium, and lysozyme levels may be elevated but are often normal in mild disease or sarcoidosis with only ocular manifestations. Chest X ray or CT will assist in identifying hilar or mediastinal lymphadenopathy. An electrocardiogram should always be obtained, since conduction blocks due to cardiac sarcoidosis can be fatal. Skin testing identifying anergy to common antigens (e.g., to *Candida* or *M. tuberculosis*, the latter for individuals who have received BCG vaccination) is supportive of the diagnosis. Skin biopsy, conjunctival biopsy, bronchoalveolar lavage, transbronchial biopsy of hilar lymphaden-opathy, and pulmonary function tests may be considered in appropriate cases.
- Treatment: Topical and periocular injections of corticosteroids can control the intraocular inflammation in a majority of cases. However, oral corticosteroids and/or immunosuppressive agents may be necessary for severe intraocular inflammation or if vital organs such as the heart and central nervous system are involved
- Prognosis: Visual outcomes are generally good in the absence of glaucoma, optic disc granuloma, or central nervous system involvement

VKH Disease

VKH disease, also known as uveomeningoencephalitic syndrome, is a multi-system disorder occurring commonly in individuals of Mongoloid descent, such as Japanese and other East Asians, North and South American Indians, and certain Hispanic groups, all populations with high rates of the HLA-DR4 haplotype. The disease presents acutely with flu-like prodromal symptoms and the onset of serous retinal detachments affecting the posterior poles bilaterally followed closely by initially mild anterior segment inflammation. Untreated or inadequately treated at this stage, the retinal detachments often progress to involve the periphery and become bullous, with more severe and progressively granulomatous anterior chamber inflammation observed. Even if untreated, the serous retinal detachments will subside in most cases; however, the disease will often become chronic with persistent or recurrent choroiditis, cystoid macular edema, papillitis, and in rare instances recurrent serous retinal detachment. In addition, anterior segment complications such as iris synechia, glaucoma, and cataract can ensue. In the convalescent stage, one can observe varying degrees of "sunset glow" or generalized depigmentation of the fundus, with chorioretinal atrophic spots dotting the periphery. However, in the end stage of severe disease, widespread geographic chorioretinal atrophy as well as systemic manifestations of poliosis, alopecia, and vitiligo may develop, usually several months to a year after the onset of disease. Prompt diagnosis and initiation of treatment in the acute stage leads to good ocular outcomes, avoidance of late skin, and hair manifestations, and essentially cessation of disease. Revised international diagnostic criteria have been recently published in order to standardize nomenclature for this disorder (Table 4) (56). Frequency of inflammatory recurrences and overall duration of disease has been identified as risk factors for ocular complications and poor visual

Table 4 Revised Diagnostic Criteria for VKH Disease by the International Committee on Nomenclature

Definitions
For "complete VKH disease," criteria 1 to 5 must be present.
For "incomplete VKH disease," criteria 1 to 3 and either 4 or 5 must be present.
For "probable VKH disease" (isolated ocular disease), criteria 1 to 3 must be present.

Criteria
1. No history of penetrating ocular trauma or surgery preceding the initial onset of uveitis.
2. No clinical or laboratory evidence suggestive of other ocular disease entities.
3. Bilateral ocular involvement (a or b must be met, depending on the stage of disease when the patient is examined).
   a. Early manifestations of disease
      (1) Evidence of diffuse choroiditis (with or without anterior uveitis, vitreous inflammatory reaction, or optic disc hyperemia), which may manifest as one of the following:
         (a) Focal areas of subretinal fluid, or
         (b) Bullous serous retinal detachments
      (2) With equivocal fundus findings, both of the following must be present as well:
         (a) Focal areas of delay in choroidal perfusion, multifocal areas of pinpoint leakage, large placoid areas of hyperfluorescence, pooling within subretinal fluid, and optic nerve staining by fluorescein angiography
         (b) Diffuse choroidal thickening, without evidence of posterior scleritis by ultra-sonography
   b. Late manifestations of disease
      (1) History suggestive of prior presence of findings from 3a, and either both (2) and (3) below, or multiple signs from (3)
      (2) Ocular depigmentation
         (a) Sunset glow fundus, or
         (b) Sugiura's sign
      (3) Other ocular signs
         (a) Nummular chorioretinal depigmented scars, or
         (b) Retinal pigment epithelium clumping and/or migration, or
         (c) Recurrent or chronic anterior uveitis

(Continued)

Table 4 Revised Diagnostic Criteria for VKH Disease by the International Committee on Nomenclature (*Continued*)

---

4. Neurological/auditory findings (may have resolved by time of examination)
   a. Meningismus (malaise, fever, headache, nausea, abdominal pain, neck or back stiffness, or a combination of these factors; headache alone is not sufficient to meet definition of meningismus, however), or
   b. Tinnitus, or
   c. Cerebrospinal fluid pleocytosis
5. Integumentary findings (not preceding onset of central nervous system or ocular disease)
   a. Alopecia, or
   b. Poliosis, or
   c. Vitiligo

Abbreviation: VKH, Vogt-Koyanagi-Harada.
Source: Adapted from Ref. 56

outcomes (57). Systemic corticosteroids are widely accepted as the drug of choice in the treatment of VKH disease; however, there is lack of consensus regarding the appropriate initial dose and route of administration (oral vs. intravenous). One international, retrospective, multicenter study showed no difference between oral versus intravenous therapy in the initial corticosteroid administration (58); however, the follow-up was variable and relatively short.

- Presenting symptoms: Prodromal flu-like symptoms, including fever, malaise, headache, meningismus, and/or tinnitus commonly occur days to a couple of weeks prior to the onset of ocular symptoms of red eye, decreased vision, and/or metamorphopsia
- Medical history/demographic associations: East Asian, North and South American Indian, or Hispanic descent
- Ocular signs (Fig. 23): Always bilateral by current diagnostic criteria (Table 3). *Anterior*: Acute stage—ciliary conjunctival injection followed by mild anterior chamber cells, then progressively granulomatous anterior segment inflammation. *Posterior*: Acute stage—serous retinal detachments affecting the posterior pole (Fig. 10), bullous retinal detachments, choroidal white lesions, papillitis, and rarely choroidal detachment. Mild vitritis may be present. Convalescent stage—generalized sunset glow fundus depigmentation, nummular chorioretinal atrophic scars in periphery, geographic chorioretinal atrophy, pigment migration occasionally in a crescent pattern in the periphery (scimitar sign), peripapillary atrophy, optic atrophy, subretinal fibrosis, CNV. *Other*: Perilimbal depigmentation (Sugiura's sign) may be observed in the convalescent stage
- Systemic signs: Poliosis, alopecia, and/or vitiligo occurring as late manifestations in untreated or severe disease

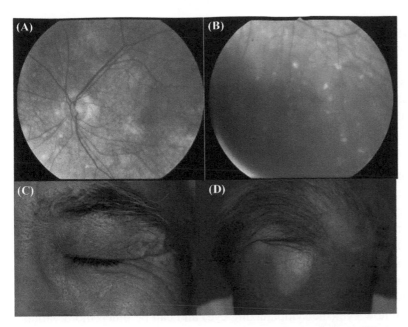

Figure 23 Composite feature of Vogt-Koyanagi-Harada disease. (**A**) A sunset glow fundus appearance during the convalescent stage. Note the granular pigmentary changes in the top of the photograph, indicative of a generalized pigment migration in addition to the depigmentation of the RPE and choroid. (**B**) Multifocal nummular chorioretinal atrophic scars in the peripheral retina during the convalescent stage. (**C**) Vitiligo around the eyes and (**D**) the scalp in chronic inflammation.

- Workup: Fluorescein angiography in the acute phase will reveal pinpoint leakages at the RPE level in early images, followed by fluorescein pooling and disc staining or leakage in late images. Cerebrospinal fluid analysis will reveal pleocytosis in up to 100% of patients in the acute phase of disease (59). B scan ultrasonography may be helpful in identifying choroidal thickening in atypical presentations or when there is poor fundus visualization. HLA-DR4 positivity and indocyanine green angiography (60) features may support the diagnosis
- Treatment: Topical and systemic corticosteroids, the latter administered in high doses of at least 1 to 1.5 mg/kg/day equivalent of prednisolone, if given orally. Intravenous treatment often involves initially administering 200 mg/day prednisolone to 1000 mg/day methylprednisolone given for three days ("pulse" dosing), followed by oral corticosteroids. Repeat pulse therapy may be considered after one week if evidence for active inflammation persists by fluorescein angiography. Oral and topical corticosteroids are tapered slowly over four to six months depending on the severity of initial disease. Immunosuppressive drugs such as

cyclosporine should be used as steroid-sparing agents in patients with severe disease who are likely to require prolonged treatment (>6 months) and in patients with relative contraindications to corticosteroid therapy such as those with diabetes mellitus

- Prognosis: Visual outcomes good with initiation of adequate treatment in the acute phase

Sympathetic Ophthalmia

Sympathetic ophthalmia (SO) is a disorder closely related to VKH disease, with similar ocular manifestations that occur in individuals with a history of penetrating ocular trauma or intraocular surgery. A prospective study has shown that SO in the modern era is most likely related to previous vitrectomy, particularly for retinal detachment (61) or scleral buckling, and occurs usually within one year of the surgical procedure. SO has been known to occur after skin trauma such as burns and (Nd: YAG) laser iridotomy, although these are rare. Intraocular inflammation is usually more severe in the eye with the history of trauma or surgery (the exciting eye) than in the fellow eye (the sympathizing eye) and can be much more variable when compared to VKH disease. For example, choroidal detachment with mild anterior segment inflammation may be the initial manifestation in a sympathizing eye. Detection of intraocular inflammation in the exciting eye may be difficult to distinguish from postoperative inflammation. Prodromal symptoms similar to those commonly noted in VKH disease may occur, but they are unusual in SO, as are the late skin and hair manifestations of alopecia, poliosis, and vitiligo. However, both SO and VKH disease share a strong association with the HLA-DR4 haplotype (62), and therefore may have a higher incidence in the same ethnic groups in which VKH disease commonly occurs. Early diagnosis can lead to good visual outcomes; however, since SO is a rare disease with great variability in initial manifestations, it is often not suspected in the early stages.

- Presenting symptoms: Red eye, floaters, decreased vision in exciting eye only, the sympathizing eye only, or both
- Medical history/demographic associations: Previous penetrating ocular trauma or surgery
- Ocular signs (Fig. 24): Always bilateral, with no one pattern of manifestations. *Anterior*: Mild-to-moderate usually granulomatous anterior segment inflammation. Anterior segment inflammation may be the only manifestation of SO. *Posterior*: Acute stage—mild vitritis, serous retinal detachment, choroidal detachment, multifocal choroidal white lesions, papillitis. Convalescent stage—generalized fundus depigmentation, nummular chorioretinal atrophic scars, geographic chorioretinal

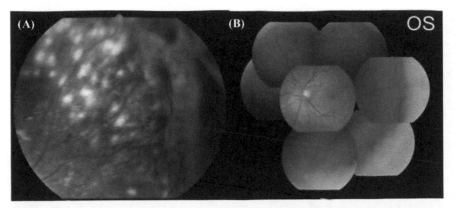

Figure 24 Fundal color photographs demonstrating features of sympathetic ophthalmia. (A) Multiple, large nummular chorioretinal scars are observed in the periphery of the *exciting* eye of the a patient with sympathetic ophthalmia. (B) Choroidal detachment for 360° was observed in the *sympathizing* eye of a different patient. The exciting eye had a history of uneventful scleral buckling for rhegmatogenous retinal detachment.

> atrophy, pigment migration, peripapillary and/or optic atrophy, CNV, subretinal fibrosis.
> - Systemic signs: Usually none
> - Workup: Fluorescein angiography to delineate choroidal inflammation. B scan ultrasonography, CSF examination, HLA-DR4 testing may be considered as appropriate (see sect. "VKH Disease")
> - Treatment: Enucleation or evisceration of the exciting eye should only be considered if painful and blind. Treatment is the same as for VKH disease with the administration of topical and systemic corticosteroids (see sect. "VKH Disease")
> - Prognosis: Visual outcomes may be good, depending on baseline visual function prior to the onset of SO

Systemic Lupus Erythematosis

Systemic lupus erythematosis (SLE) is a systemic vasculitic disorder characterized by the development of a variety of autoantibodies, most notably various antinuclear antibodies and antiphospholipid antibodies, and circulating immune complexes. The disease is most common in young to middle-aged women who may experience systemic symptoms of fatigue, fever, malaise, and/or arthralgias before ocular symptoms develop. The disease can eventually cause arthritis, glomerulonephritis, pericarditis, pleurisy, various hematological abnormalities

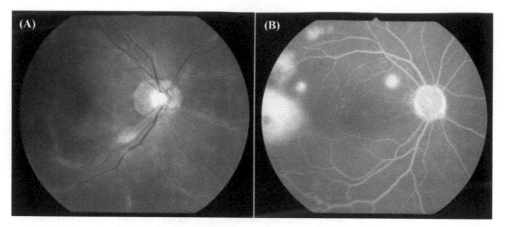

Figure 25 Fundal color photograph and flourescein angiogram of retinal features in SLE. (**A**) Severe retinal vasculitis involving both veins and arteries. (**B**) Fluorescein angiography of another patient shows points of dye leakage with pooling in areas of focal retinal detachment.

such as leukopenia and thrombocytopenia, splenomegaly, and numerous central nervous system abnormalities.

- Presenting symptoms: Decreased vision, ocular involvement may be asymptomatic
- Medical history/demographic associations: Adult women
- Ocular signs (Fig. 25): When intraocular inflammation is present, it is usually bilateral, albeit frequently asymmetric in severity. *Anterior*: No anterior segment intraocular inflammation. *Posterior*: Absence of vitritis; multifocal choroiditis, retinal vasculitis, serous retinal detachment, optic neuropathy. *Other*: Keratoconjunctivitis sicca, peripheral ulcerative keratitis, scleritis
- Systemic signs: Fever, "butterfly" malar rash, discoid rash, Raynaud's phenomenon, alopecia, oral ulceration
- Workup: Elevated erythrocyte sedimentation rate and/or C-reactive protein, and the presence of antinuclear antibodies and antiphospholipid antibodies would support the diagnosis of SLE. Serum creatinine and urinalysis should be examined to screen for renal disease
- Treatment: Successful control of systemic disease using corticosteroids, immunosuppressive drugs, and/or biological agents usually results in control of the intraocular inflammation
- Prognosis: Visual outcomes are relatively good unless optic atrophy ensues

Multiple Sclerosis

Multiple sclerosis (MS) is a demyelinating disease of the central nervous system that usually presents to the ophthalmologist with optic neuritis or internuclear ophthalmoplegia and other gaze palsies. MS can also cause mild intraocular inflammation, usually in the form of a peripheral retinal periphlebitis. It is unclear whether this feature is associated temporally with the development of optic neuritis. However, periphlebitis is observed in roughly one-quarter of patients with optic neuritis, and patients with optic neuritis in the setting of periphlebitis may have a higher incidence of progression to clinically diagnosed MS (63).

- Presenting symptoms: Floaters, decreased vision
- Medical history/demographic associations: History of neurological abnormalities
- Ocular signs: PSII (other than optic neuritis) may be unilateral or bilateral and not dissimilar to many cases with intermediate uveitis. *Anterior*: Mild anterior segment intraocular inflammation. *Posterior*: Anterior vitritis, pars planitis, periphlebitis, or venous sheathing in the peripheral retina. *Other*: Optic neuritis, internuclear ophthalmoplegia, skew deviation, cranial nerve palsies, nystagmus
- Systemic signs: Neurological deficits may be present
- Workup: Cerebrospinal fluid examination may be positive for oligoclonal bands. Brain MRI may show active plaques in the periventricular regions
- Treatment: Topical and/or periocular injections of corticosteroids are generally adequate to control active intraocular inflammation. Peripheral periphlebitis alone does not require treatment, although more severe posterior segment inflammation may benefit from immunosuppression. Systemic interferon-β therapy may be used to treat the underlying MS
- Prognosis: Visual outcomes usually good for intraocular inflammation unless optic neuritis occurs

Frosted Branch Angiitis

Frosted branch angiitis is a term used to describe the severe retinal vasculitis, particularly affecting the veins, which can accompany CMV retinitis (64) and many other infections such as tuberculosis and syphilis, as well as presumed autoinflammatory processes such as systemic lupus erythematosus. Regardless of any primary infection, the pathogenesis of frosted branch angiitis is believed to be autoinflammatory in nature.

- Presenting symptoms: Decreased vision, floaters, photophobia
- Medical history/demographic associations: AIDS, immunosuppression, tuberculosis, syphilis, systemic lupus erythematosus, other autoinflammatory disorders
- Ocular signs: Bilateral in roughly three-fourths of patients. *Anterior*: Mild-to-moderate anterior segment inflammation. *Posterior*: Mild-to-moderate vitritis, prominent perivascular sheathing, with or without retinal hemorrhages, retinitis consistent with CMV infection, papillitis

- Systemic signs: None specific to frosted branch angiitis
- Workup: Consider PCR analysis of aqueous or vitreous if necessary to rule out active CMV or other infection
- Treatment: Systemic corticosteroids may be considered, but specific treatment must be carried out for any primary infection if present
- Prognosis: Variable

Presumed Autoinflammatory Diseases, Without Systemic Manifestations

The following section describes presumed autoinflammatory ocular disorders that occur in the absence of systemic manifestations. Unlike those with systemic manifestations, these are not necessarily bilateral. There is much overlap and confusion with the clinical delineation of many of these disorders, also referred to collectively as white dot syndromes, complicating research in this field and the ability of clinicians to treat patients. In fact, a definitive diagnosis is probably less important than determining whether sight is under threat. Autoimmunity to retinal antigens has been shown in some of these conditions, however, the relationship with "so-called" autoimmune retinopathy is not clear. Studies in animal models have shown that many of the different clinical syndromes can be mimicked by immunization to a restricted set of retinal or ocular antigens (see chap. 6). For the practicing physician, determination of the threat to sight is the key to good management.

Multifocal Evanescent White Dot Syndrome

MEWDS is an uncommon, transient, unilateral, self-limiting disorder of acute onset usually occurring in young adult women and has a benign natural course. Some patients may recall flu-like symptoms preceding the onset of visual disturbance. The fundus changes in MEWDS appear to be limited to the outer retina and the RPE. Many specialists consider MEWDS to be one presentation within a spectrum of disorders, including acute idiopathic blind spot enlargement (AIBSE), acute zonal occult outer retinopathy (AZOOR), acute annular outer retinopathy (AAOR), and acute macular neuroretinopathy (AMN) (65), and these are described in the next section.

- Presenting symptoms: Photophobia, flashing lights, decreased vision, scotoma
- Medical history/demographic associations: Flu-like illness one to two weeks prior. Most common in women aged 20 to 40 years

- Ocular signs: Usually unilateral. *Anterior*: No anterior segment inflammation. *Posterior*: Acute phase—mild vitreous cells, multiple white spots with rather indistinct borders at the level of the RPE in the posterior pole to mid-periphery (see Fig. 6; also see Fig. 18 of chap. 2), mild papillitis or optic disc edema. All changes resolve over weeks. Mild retinal vascular sheathing may be present. Convalescent phase—fine granular appearance of the macula. CNV is a rare complication. *Other*: A relative afferent pupillary defect may be present in the acute phase that resolves completely
- Systemic signs: Usually none
- Workup: Fluorescein angiography will show early punctate hyperfluorescence with late staining of lesions, with or without mild optic disc staining. Indocyanine green angiography will show hypofluorescence of lesions. Goldmann visual field may reveal an enlarged blind spot and electroretinography (ERG) may show generalized reduced amplitudes, both changes that resolve
- Treatment: Not necessary unless CNV develops
- Prognosis: Usually good

MEWDS-Related Outer Retinopathies (AIBSE, AZOOR, AAOR, AMN)

All of the MEWDS-related outer retinopathies are rare, occur somewhat more commonly in young women, and often show evidence of blind spot enlargement in the acute phase of disease. Similar to MEWDS, all are believed to involve dysfunction of the photoreceptors and RPE. As mentioned above, there is considerable overlap of clinical features of these disorders, and the nomenclature and diagnostic criteria for these disorders remain under considerable debate. Thus, although these entities, including MEWDS, have "names" attached to them, they may merely represent variations on a spectrum of the same disease, albeit with possible differences in triggering etiology. Furthermore, progression of visual loss has been reported, with subsequent control on immunosuppression (66). Therefore, assuming that the pathogenesis involves an autoinflammatory process, immunosuppressive therapy should be considered in patients with progressive disease.

- AIBSE is characterized by symptoms of unilateral photopsia and an enlarged blind spot on visual field testing. Funduscopy may show mild disc hyperemia but may also be entirely normal. Unlike MEWDS, it is said that the visual field abnormality in AIBSE may not recover completely. However, a long-term follow-up study has shown that many cases initially diagnosed as AIBSE can be reclassified later as having either MEWDS, one of the related disease entities below, or what has been poorly termed pseudo-presumed ocular histoplasmosis syndrome (67), most cases of which were probably multifocal choroiditis with panuveitis (MCP).

- AZOOR is characterized by photopsia and rapid onset of large zones of outer retinal dysfunction in one or both eyes. Only minimal funduscopic change may be visible in the acute phase, with the gradual development of RPE atrophy and narrowing of retinal vessels in the zone of dysfunction (68). ERG and visual field abnormalities associated with the retinal dysfunction are usually permanent.
- AAOR is characterized by the appearance of a whitish ring surrounding the disc or in the macula that gradually enlarges then resolves over days to weeks (Fig. 26), often in only one eye with reduced vision (69). However, multifocal ERG may reveal reduced macular function in both eyes, and the disease can be progressive and require immunosuppression (66).
- AMN is characterized by wedge-shaped, grayish to reddish brown lesions at the level of the outer retina in the macula, usually in both eyes of young patients complaining of mild decreased vision after a flu-like illness. The lesions and vision improve spontaneously over weeks to months, usually with no sequelae.

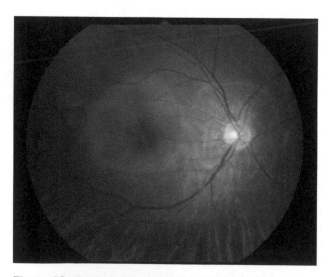

Figure 26 Fundus color photograph of AAOR. Whitish ring formation around the disc and in the macula of this patient diagnosed with AAOR. *Abbreviation*: AAOR, acute annular outer retinopathy. (With permission, Archives of Ophthalmology, American Medical Association.)

Acute Posterior Multifocal Placoid Pigment Epitheliopathy

APMPPE is usually a bilateral, self-limited disorder occurring in adults often after a flu-like illness. The disease is characterized by creamy-white placoid lesions, larger in size than MEWDS lesions, which appear in the posterior pole at the level of the RPE and resolve over a period of weeks. Complete visual recovery occurs in the majority of patients. Most patients develop varying degrees of chorioretinal atrophy in the convalescent phase. However, in rare cases, severe pigmented scarring with poor visual outcome can be observed similar to that seen in serpiginous choroidopathy, a disease entity with which there is some overlap of features (see sect. "serpiginous choroidopathy"). Rarely, APMPPE may be associated with dermal vasculitis, nephropathy, cerebral vasculitis, meningoence-phalopathy, and thyroiditis. APMPPE has been reported in association with serous retinal detachment (70), but these cases must be carefully differentiated from VKH disease by systemic symptoms and signs.

- Presenting symptoms: Decreased central vision, photopsia
- Medical history/demographic associations: Recent flu-like illness
- Ocular signs (Fig. 27): Usually bilateral. *Anterior*: No anterior segment inflammation. *Posterior*: Mild vitritis, multiple creamy-white placoid lesions in the posterior pole that evolve into patchy areas of chorioretinal atrophy
- Systemic signs: Usually none; however, neurological abnormalities may be present with CNS involvement

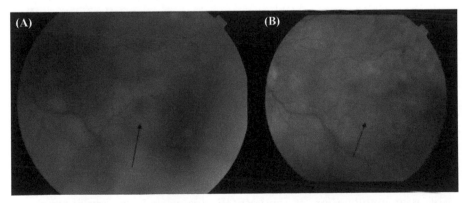

Figure 27 Fundus color photographs of APMPPE. (**A**) Acute phase showing classic deep creamy placoid lesions (*arrow*) and (**B**) evolving into atrophic granular appearance (*arrow*). *Abbreviation*: APMPPE, acute posterior multifocal placoid pigment epitheliopathy.

- Workup: Fluorescein angiography shows early hypofluorescence and late hyperfluorescence of lesions. Indocyanine green angiography demonstrates hypofluorescence of lesions
- Treatment: None for the ocular manifestations, although systemic corticosteroids may be appropriate for neurological involvement
- Prognosis: Visual outcomes usually good

Serpiginous Choroidopathy

Serpiginous choroidopathy (also called geographic choroiditis) is a rare, insidious, bilateral, progressive disorder characterized by recurrences of inflammation at the level of the inner choroid and RPE, gradually leading over several years to severe geographic pigmented chorioretinal scarring of the entire posterior pole. Since the disease usually starts in the peripapillary region, patients may be asymptomatic despite fairly advanced bilateral disease until the fovea of one of the eyes is involved, prompting the patient to seek ophthalmological consultation. The disease is most commonly diagnosed in older adults, and CNV may develop as a complication, limiting central vision further. Although systemic corticosteroids and immunosuppressive agents, often in combination, are used to treat serpiginous choroidopathy (71), the overall visual prognosis remains poor for this disease. Some patients show clinical features that are intermediate between APMPPE and serpiginous choroidopathy, and these cases have been referred to as relentless placoid chorioretinitis (72), highlighting our lack of knowledge into the pathogenesis of these disorders.

- Presenting symptoms: Decreased vision, metamorphopsia
- Medical history/demographic associations: Middle-aged or older adult
- Ocular signs (see Fig. 17 of chap. 2): Usually bilateral, but may be asymmetric. *Anterior*: Mild-to-no anterior segment inflammation. *Posterior*: Mild vitritis. Active lesions appear creamy-white to gray with retinal thickening, initially in the peripapillary region, often adjacent to old inactive scars. Lesions become atrophic over weeks, adding in a "serpiginous" manner to previous geographic scars that slowly expand to involve most of the posterior pole. CNV is a common late complication
- Systemic signs: None
- Workup: Fluorescein angiography shows early hypofluorescence and late hyperfluorescence of active lesions
- Treatment: Immunosuppressive agents, often in combination with systemic corticosteroids. Photodynamic therapy or intravitreal injection of triamcinolone or an anti-VEGF agent such as ranibizumab or bevacizumab may be considered for CNV
- Prognosis: Visual outcomes are generally poor

Table 5 Birdshot Chorioretinopathy Diagnostic Criteria for Research Purposes by an International Consensus Conference

Required characteristics	1. Bilateral disease
	2. Presence of at least three peripapillary "birdshot lesions" inferior or nasal to the optic disc in one eye
	3. Low-grade anterior segment intraocular inflammation (defined as ≤1+ cells in the anterior chamber)[a]
	4. Low-grade vitreous inflammatory reaction (defined as ≤2+ vitreous haze)[b]
Supportive findings	1. HLA-A29 positivity
	2. Retinal vasculitis
	3. Cystoid macular edema
Exclusion criteria	1. Keratic precipitates
	2. Posterior synechiae
	3. Presence of infective, neoplastic, or other inflammatory diseases that can cause multifocal choroidal lesions

[a]Defined by the Standardization of Uveitis Nomenclature (SUN) Working Group (1).
[b]Defined by Nussenblatt et al. (77).
Abbreviation: HLA, human leukocyte antigen.
Source: From Ref. 76.

Birdshot Chorioretinopathy

Birdshot chorioretinopathy is an uncommon bilateral disorder occurring in middle-aged Caucasian adults, and is strongly associated with the HLA-A29 haplotype. The disease is characterized by distinctive creamy-white oval lesions deep to the sensory retina oriented in a radiating pattern from the disc into the periphery, with mild papillitis but usually very little anterior segment or vitreous inflammation. Gradual loss of vision over years occurs due to chronic cystoid macular edema (73) with subsequent macular atrophy. Color vision testing and ERG appear to be useful in monitoring disease progression since clinically observable features and visual acuity are not reliable indicators of disease activity (73–75). CNV may occur as a late complication. An international consensus conference has published research criteria for the diagnosis of birdshot chorioretinopathy (Table 5) (76). The aggressive use of systemic immunosuppressive agents and corticosteroids may prolong visual function to some extent (78); however, overall visual prognosis remains poor for this disease.

- Presenting symptoms: Decreased vision, floaters
- Medical history/demographic associations: Middle-aged or older Caucasian individuals

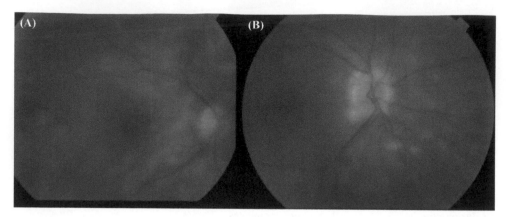

Figure 28 Fundal color photographs of birdshot chorioretinopathy. (**A**) Early deep retinal/choroidal lesions around the optic nerve. (**B**) Even in the chronic stages, deep lesions do not develop pigmentation.

- Ocular signs (Fig. 28): Always bilateral by current diagnostic criteria (76). *Anterior*: Mild-to-no anterior segment inflammation. Keratic precipitates and posterior synechia are not observed. *Posterior*: Mild vitritis, multiple creamy-white, nonpigmented, oval, or round lesions at the level of the choroid, clustered around the optic disc radiating to the periphery. New lesions develop while old lesions evolve into atrophic spots. Cystoid macular edema, optic disc edema, and retinal vasculitis are common. CNV, optic atrophy, and macular atrophy occur as late complications
- Systemic signs: None
- Workup: Fluorescein angiography shows early hypofluorescence and late hyperfluorescence of some but not all funduscopically visible choroidal lesions. Indocyanine green angiography may reveal hypofluorescence of lesions. HLA-A29 testing is positive in up to 96% of patients (79). ERG shows reduced amplitude and increased latency of the b-wave (80) and ERG parameters appear to correlate with disease activity (75). Color vision testing may be abnormal even in eyes with good visual acuity (73)
- Treatment: Immunosuppressive agents, often in combination with systemic corticosteroids
- Prognosis: Long-term visual outcomes are poor

Multifocal Choroiditis with Panuveitis

MCP is a somewhat loosely used term for a poorly defined clinical entity featuring the bilateral development of multiple choroidal white lesions that evolve into pigmented atrophic scars in the presence of moderate vitritis. MCP is closely related to PIC and diffuse subretinal fibrosis (DSF) syndrome, both of which are covered in the next section. All three disorders occur most commonly in young women who are myopic, although it is said that the age of onset is youngest for PIC. Furthermore, some patients previously reported as having pseudo-presumed ocular histoplasmosis syndrome (i.e., ocular histoplasmosis with vitritis) were likely cases of MCP (67). However, one must remember that a wide variety of infectious, autoinflammatory, and even neoplastic disorders can manifest as a multifocal choroiditis with vitreous and/or anterior chamber cells (see differential diagnosis list for choroiditis). Therefore, when considering the diagnosis of MCP, one must be careful to rule out other possible causes to explain the clinical features, particularly in patients with systemic symptoms such as fever, malaise, or arthritis. In general, MCP is chronic and rather indolent in progression, whereas infectious, autoinflammatory, and neoplastic disorders will generally worsen more quickly. However, CNV has been reported in 22% of eyes with MCP, leading to visual loss (81). Other complications reducing vision include epiretinal membrane and cystoid macular edema.

- Presenting symptoms: Decreased vision, metamorphopsia, floaters, photopsia
- Medical history/demographic associations: Young, myopic women
- Ocular signs (Fig. 29): Usually bilateral, but may be asymmetric in severity. *Anterior*: Mild anterior segment inflammation. *Posterior*: Mild-to-moderate vitritis, yellowish or grayish lesions at the level of RPE

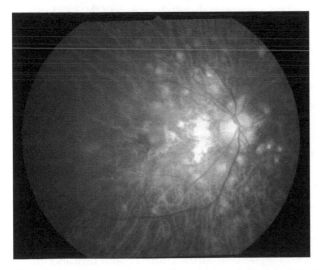

Figure 29 Fundal color photograph demonstrating clinical features of multifocal choroiditis. Multifocal chorioretinal atrophic scars and peripapillary atrophy are characteristic of multifocal choroiditis and panuveitis. (Note the secondary choroidal neovascularization in the fovea).

or inner choroid, varying greatly in size, usually in the peripapillary region. Lesions evolve into round, pigmented chorioretinal spots that may appear similar to ocular histoplasmosis lesions. Papillitis, cystoid macular edema, and/or epiretinal membrane may be present. CNV may occur as a late complication and result in a poor visual outcome

- Systemic signs: None
- Workup: Fluorescein angiography shows early hypofluorescence and late hyperfluorescence of new lesions. Indocyanine green angiography shows hypofluorescence of lesions and may show more lesions that can be observed on funduscopic examination. Full-field ERG or multifocal ERG may show reduced amplitudes. Goldmann visual field testing will show scotomas corresponding to affected areas of retina and in many cases an enlarged blind spot. Specific tests to rule out syphilis, tuberculosis, sarcoidosis, Lyme disease, and birdshot chorioretinopathy should be considered
- Treatment: Topical corticosteroids for anterior segment inflammation. Periocular corticosteroid injections may be used for severe vitritis and for new macular lesions or cystoid macular edema. Systemic corticosteroids and/or immunosuppression may also be considered for chronic or recurrent disease. Photodynamic therapy or intravitreal injection of triamcinolone or an anti-VEGF agent such a ranibizumab or bevacizumab may be used to treat CNV
- Prognosis: Visual outcomes vary depending on foveal involvement either by choroiditis, macular edema, epiretinal membrane, or CNV (81)

PIC and DSF Syndrome

PIC and DSF syndrome may be different manifestations of the same disorder and both are closely related to MCP in that the development of multifocal choroiditis is the predominant feature (82). However, while eyes with MCP characteristically have at least moderate vitritis, PIC and DSF syndrome are not associated with significant vitreous inflammation. PIC, like MCP, occurs in young otherwise healthy, myopic women who often present with vague complaints of blurred vision, photopsia, and central scotomas. Funduscopy will reveal active yellow spots in the choroid of the posterior pole that atrophy over time and usually do not recur. However, CNV may develop as a late complication in PIC (Fig. 30). DSF syndrome is much more rare than PIC and occurs in the same demographic group of patients. Eyes diagnosed with DSF syndrome show chorioretinal lesions similar to those seen in PIC, but in association with progressive subretinal fibrosis in one

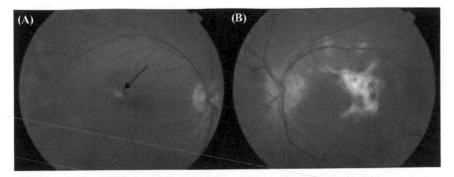

Figure 30 Fundal color photographs of patient with PIC and subretinal fibrosis. (**A**) Early choroidal neovascular membrane (*arrow*) and (**B**) fellow eye displaying chronic course of PIC complicated by central subretinal fibrosis. *Abbreviation*: PIC, punctate inner choroidopathy.

or both eyes. As in PIC, other possible infective, autoinflammatory or neoplastic causes of multifocal choroiditis should be ruled out.

- Presenting symptoms: Decreased vision, photopsia, central scotoma
- Medical history/demographic associations: Young, myopic women
- Ocular signs: Usually bilateral but may be asymmetric in severity. *Anterior*: No anterior segment inflammation. *Posterior*: Mild-to-no vitritis, multiple yellowish spots at the level of RPE or inner choroid, usually clustered in the macula, sometimes in association with mild subretinal fluid. Lesions atrophy over time, often with pigmentation and distinct round borders. CNV may occur as a late complication in PIC. Eyes with DSF syndrome develop progressive pigmented subretinal scarring
- Systemic signs: None
- Workup: Same as in PIC
- Treatment: Eyes with PIC usually only require treatment for secondary CNV, with either photodynamic therapy, periocular injection of cortico-steroids or intravitreal injection of an anti-VEGF agent. In eyes with DSF syndrome and active (evolving) subretinal fibrosis, aggressive treatment with periocular corticosteroid injections and/or systemic immunosup-pressive treatment may halt the progression of scarring
- Prognosis: Visual outcomes vary depending on foveal involvement either by CNV or subretinal fibrosis

Pars Planitis

There exists some controversy over this terminology; however, the current consensus is to use the disease name "pars planitis" to denote intermediate uveitis of unknown etiology, i.e., after ruling out the possible differential diseases as listed in the first section of this chapter. Some uveitis specialists prefer the term "idiopathic intermediate uveitis," particularly since much of the older literature lumped together intermediate uveitis of a variety of etiologies together into pars planitis. Regardless, the hallmark of pars planitis is chronic anterior vitritis in the presence of exudates or snowbanking over the pars plana and/or peripheral retina. There is often nearby peripheral retinal vasculitis. The major diseases to consider in such a setting are HTLV-1 uveitis, Lyme disease, syphilis, toxocariasis, sarcoidosis, MS, and intraocular lymphoma. In the absence of evidence for such diseases, the term pars planitis may be used and this disease entity may account for up to 25% of patients in some uveitis specialty clinics in North America and Europe (83). As it turns out, patients with pars planitis appear to share certain epidemiological features, such as a higher incidence in children and young adults, and in Caucasian populations. However, it should also be noted that many patients initially given a diagnosis of pars planitis, later develop MS (84) or other systemic disease. The major difficulty in treatment of this disease is the development of secondary cystoid macular edema. Cataract is a frequent complication.

- Presenting symptoms: Painless blurring of vision, floaters, photophobia
- Medical history/demographic associations: Children and young adults, common in Caucasians, rare in Asian and African populations
- Ocular signs: *Anterior*: Mild anterior chamber cells usually without iris synechia. *Posterior*: Mild-to-severe cells in the anterior vitreous with snowballs, exudates or snowbanking over the pars plana, and/or peripheral retina (see Fig. 2 of chap. 2), with a chronic, "smoldering" clinical course. There is often evidence of peripheral retinal vasculitis such as vascular sheathing. Cystoid macular edema and cataract are common complications. Epiretinal membrane formation, retinal neo-vascularization, disc neovascularization, and even retinal detachment (exudative, tractional or rhegmatogenous) may also occur
- Systemic signs: None
- Workup: Optical coherence tomography will help one to assess cystoid macular edema. Fluorescein angiography is useful to delineate cystoid macular edema, peripheral nonperfusion and possible neovascularization. Of course, specific tests should be performed to rule out HTLV-1 uveitis, Lyme disease, syphilis, toxocariasis, sarcoidosis, MS, and intraocular lymphoma
- Treatment: The goal is to control inflammation in order to avoid the many complications. This may include topical, periocular, intravitreal, and/or systemic corticosteroid administration. Cryotherapy or panretinal photocoagulation may be considered if neovascularization is not

responsive to corticosteroid treatment. Immunosuppressive agents such as cyclosporine should be considered if prolonged systemic treatment is required. Cataract extraction with intraocular lens implantation is generally successful. Vitrectomy may be required for severe vitreous debris or membranes, refractory cystoid macular edema, epiretinal membrane, or retinal detachment

- Prognosis: Usually good except in cases of prolonged cystoid macular edema or retinal detachment (84)

Neoplastic Disease

A section on neoplastic disease is included in this text because of the difficulty in differentiating intraocular lymphoma from traditional "uveitis," and because the treatment and/or follow-up of this disorder often falls into the hands of the uveitis specialist. Intraocular lymphoma may be particularly difficult to distinguish from ocular sarcoidosis.

Intraocular Lymphoma

Intraocular lymphoma may be observed either as a manifestation of primary central nervous system lymphoma (PCNSL, a large cell non-Hodgkin's lymphoma), or less commonly as metastatic disease from systemic lymphomas such as non-Hodgkin's lymphoma, Hodgkin's lymphoma, Burkitt's lymphoma, and mycosis fungoides. The former is characterized by prominent vitritis or multiple small sub-RPE infiltrates, while the latter often presents with multiple large choroidal infiltrates. Both situations can be mistaken for intraocular inflammatory disorders, particularly sarcoidosis, but also tuberculosis, syphilis, Lyme disease, SO, MCP, *Pneumocystis* or *M. avium-intracellulare* infection, and other metastatic cancer. In general, intraocular lymphoma will ultimately progress in the absence of cancer treatment, while a disease such as sarcoidosis will respond well to local corticosteroid therapy. An elevated interleukin (IL)-10 to IL-6 ratio in vitreous samples would suggest neoplasia rather than inflammation (85), and cell surface marker studies and/or PCR testing may allow the identification of monoclonal proliferation of cells (86). Intraocular lymphoma is observed most commonly in patients aged 50 years or older, but may also occur in younger individuals with AIDS or on immunosuppressive therapy for organ transplantation or autoinflammatory disease. Intraocular lymphoma in the absence of systemic disease is termed primary intraocular lymphoma (PIOL, also formerly called reticulum cell sarcoma), and portends the eventual development of PCNSL over years in the vast majority of patients. Conversely, roughly 20% of patients

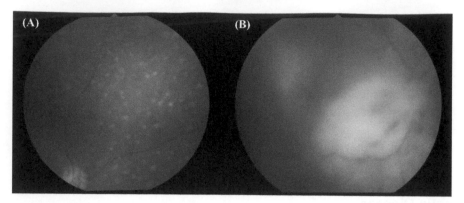

Figure 31 Fundal color photographs demonstrating varying features of intraocular lymphoma. (A) Multiple, small, discrete sub-RPE white lesions were observed in this patient with recurrent intraocular lymphoma as a manifestation of primary central nervous system lymphoma. (B) Large areas of choroidal infiltration associated with retinal hemorrhages were observed in this patient who was later diagnosed with intraocular lymphoma based on cytological examination of vitreous specimens. *Abbreviation*: RPE, retinal pigment epithelium.

initially diagnosed with nonocular PCNSL develop ocular involvement at some time (86). Overall life expectancy for PCNSL is poor. Clinical outcomes for other systemic lymphomas depend on the cell type, with cure rates being fairly high for Hodgkin's lymphoma, but rather low for non-Hodgkin's lymphoma.

- Presenting symptoms: Floaters, decreased vision
- Medical history/demographic associations: Middle-aged or elderly individuals, AIDS, immunosuppression
- Ocular signs (Fig. 31): Bilateral in over 80%. *Anterior*: Mild anterior chamber cells may be present. *Posterior*: Mild-to-severe vitritis, small multifocal sub-RPE white lesions, large areas of choroidal infiltrates, retinal vasculitis, optic disc infiltration
- Systemic signs: Fever, weight loss, malaise may be present
- Workup: Gadolinium-enhanced brain MRI and cerebrospinal fluid examination to look for CNS involvement. Diagnostic vitrectomy for cytology, IL-10 and IL-6 measurements, immunohistochemistry of cell surface markers, and/or PCR to identify specific gene rearrangements may be considered
- Treatment: Eye and/or brain radiation therapy, with or without systemic chemotherapy. Limited experience has shown that isolated PIOL may be successfully controlled with intravitreal methotrexate injections (87)
- Prognosis: Visual outcomes vary depending on the location and degree of fundus involvement

SUMMARY

The major diagnostic dilemmas of the clinician were presented in an attempt to provide an accessible reference manual for on-the-spot consultations of PSII. A general list of possible diseases can be generated based on the predominant clinical features. This list can then be narrowed down based on clues in the history, symptoms, ocular features, and systemic findings in the patient, allowing the clinician to proceed with a tailored approach to ancillary testing. Treatments for specific disease entities depend largely on the particular patient; however, overall guidelines are provided in chapters 4 and 5.

REFERENCES

1. Jabs DA, Nussenblatt RB, Rosenbaum JT. Standardization of uveitis nomenclature for reporting clinical data. Results of the first international workshop. Standardization of Uveitis Nomenclature (SUN) Working Group. Am J Ophthalmol 2005; 140:509–516.

2. Ganatra JB, Chandler D, Santos C, et al. Viral causes of the acute retinal necrosis syndrome. Am J Ophthalmol 2000; 129:166–172.

3. Silverstein BE, Conrad D, Margolis TP, et al. Cytomegalovirus-associated acute retinal necrosis syndrome. Am J Ophthlamol 1997; 123:257–258.

4. Moshfeghi DM, Dodds EM, Couto CA, et al. Diagnostic approaches to severe, atypical toxoplasmosis mimicking acute retinal necrosis. Ophthalmology 2004; 111:716–725.

5. Holland GN, Executive Committee of the American Uveitis Society. Standard diagnostic criteria for the acute retinal necrosis syndrome. Am J Ophthalmol 1994; 117:663–666.

6. de Boer JH, Verhagen C, Bruinenberg M, et al. Serologic and polymerase chain reaction analysis of intraocular fluids in the diagnosis of infectious uveitis. Am J Ophthalmol 1996; 12:650–658.

7. Engstrom RE, Holland GH, Margolis TP, et al. The progressive outer retinal necrosis syndrome: a variant of necrotizing herpetic retinopathy in patients with AIDS. Ophthalmology 1994; 101:1488–1502.

8. Kashiwase M, Sata T, Yamauchi Y, et al. Progressive outer retinal necrosis caused by herpes simplex virus type 1 in a patient with acquired immunodeficiency syndrome. Ophthalmology 2000; 107:790–794.

9. Kempen JH, Min YI, Freeman WR, et al. Risk of immune recovery uveitis in patients with AIDS and cytomegalovirus retinitis. Ophthalmology 2006; 113:684–694.

10. Song MK, Azen SP, Buley A, et al. Effect of anti-cytomegalovirus therapy on the incidence of immune recovery uveitis in AIDS patients with healed cytomegalovirus retinitis. Am J Ophthlamol 2003; 136:696–702.

11. Schrier RD, Song MK, Smith IL, et al. Intaocular viral and immune pathogenesis of immune recovery uveitis in patients with healed cytomegalovirus retinitis. Retina 2006; 26:165–169.

12. Karavellas MP, Azen SP, MacDonald JC, et al. Immune recovery vitritis and uveitis in AIDS: clinical predictors, sequelae, and treatment outcomes. Retina 2001; 21:1–9.

13. Miserocchi E, Modorati G, Brancato R. Immune recovery uveitis in an iatrogenically immunosuppressed patient. Eur J Ophthalmol 2005; 15:510–512.

14. Jabs DA, Green WR, Fox R, et al. Ocular manifestations of acquired immune deficiency syndrome. Ophthalmology 1989; 96:1092–1099.

15. National Center for Infective Diseases Division of HIV/AIDS, Centers for Disease Control. 1993 Revised classification system for HIV infection and expanded surveillance case definition for AIDS among adolescents and adults. MMWR 1992; 41(RR-17):1–19.

16. Mochizuki M, Watanabe T, Yamaguchi K, et al. Uveitis associated with human T lymphotropic virus type I. Am J Ophthalmol 1992; 114:123–129.

17. Lim WK, Mathur R, Koh A, et al. Ocular manifestations of dengue fever. Ophthalmology 2004; 111:2057–2064.

18. Schiedler V, Scott IU, Flynn HW, et al. Culture-proven endogenous endophthalmitis: clinical features and visual acuity outcomes. Am J Ophthalmol 2004; 137:725–731.

19. Binder MI, Chua J, Kaiser PK, et al. Endogenous endophthlamitis: an 18-year review of culture-positive cases at a tertiary care center. Medicine (Baltimore) 2003; 82:87–105.

20. Okada AA, Johnson RP, Liles C, D'Amico DJ, Baker AS. Endogenous endophthalmitis: a 10 year retrospective study. Ophthalmology 1994; 101:832–838.

21. Greenwald MJ, Wohl LG, Sell CH. Metastatic bacterial endophthalmitis: a contemporary reappraisal. Surv Ophthalmol 1986; 31:81–101.

22. Wong JS, Chan TK, Lee HM, et al. Endogenous bacterial endophthalmitis: an East Asian experience and a reappraisal of a severe ocular affliction. Ophthalmology 2000; 107:1483–1491.

23. Bowyer JD, Gormley PD, Seth R, et al. Choroidal tuberculosis diagnosed by polymerase chain reaction. A clinicopathologic case report. Ophthalmology 1999; 106:290–294.

24. Otsuka M, Sekizawa K. [Significance of BCG vaccination.] Nippon Naika Gakkai Zasshi 2000; 89:916–920.

25. Mori T, Sakatani M, Yamagishi F, et al. Specific detection of tuberculosis infection: an interferon-γ-based assay using new antigens. Am J Respir Crit Care Med 2004; 170:59–64.

26. Morimura Y, Okada AA, Kawahara S, et al. Tuberculin skin testing in uveitis patients and treatment of presumed ocular tuberculosis in Japan. Ophthalmology 2002; 109:851–857.

27. Gupta V, Gupta A, Arora S, et al. Presumed tubercular serpiginous-like choroiditis; clinical presentations and management. Ophthalmology 2003; 110:1744–1749.

28. Tuberculosis Coalition for Technical Assistance. International Standards for Tuberculosis Care (ISTC). The Hague: Tuberculosis Coalition for Technical Assistance, 2006.

29. Musher DM, Baughn RE. Neurosyphilis in HIV-infected persons. N Engl J Med 1994; 331:1516–1517.

30. Mikkila HO, Seppala IJT, Viljanen MK, et al. The expanding clinical spectrum of ocular Lyme borreliosis. Ophthalmology 2000; 107:581–587.

31. Winterkorn JMS. Lyme disease: neurologic and ophthalmic manifestations. Surv Ophthalmol 1990; 35:191–204.

32. Dolan MJ, Wong MT, Regnery RL, et al. Syndrome of Rochalimaea henselae adenitis suggesting cat scratch disease. Ann Intern Med 1993; 118:331–336.

33. Kohno S, Mitsutake K, Maesaki S, et al. An evaluation of serodiagnostic tests in patients with candidemia: beta-glucan, mannan, candida antigen by Cand-Tec and D-arabinitol. Microbiol Immunol 1993; 37:207–212.

34. Suttorp-Schulten MS, Bollemeijer JG, Bos PJ, et al. Presumed ocular histoplasmosis in the Netherands: an area without histoplasmosis. Br J Ophthalmol 1997; 81:7–11.

35. Rosenfeld PJ, Saperstein DA, Bressler NM, et al., and Verteporfin in Ocular Histoplasmosis Study Group. Photodynamic therapy with verteporfin in ocular histoplasmosis: uncontrolled, open-label 2-year study. Ophthalmology 2004; 111:1725–1733.

36. Rechtman E, Allen VD, Danis RP, et al. Intravitreal triamcinolone for choroidal neovascularization in ocular histoplasmosis syndrome. Am J Ophthalmol 2003; 136:739–741.

37. Dees C, Arnold JJ, Forrester JV, et al. Immunosuppressive treatment of choroidal neovascularization associated with endogenous posterior uveitis. Arch Ophthalmol 1998; 116:1456–1461.

38. Serraino D, Puro V, Boumis E, et al. Epidemiological aspects of major opportunistic infections of the respiratory tract in persons with AIDS: Europe, 1993–2000. AIDS 2003; 17:2109–2116.

39. Rao NA, Zimmerman PL, Boyer D, et al. A clinical, histopathologic, and electron microscopic study of *Pneumocystitis carinii* choroiditis. Am J Ophthalmol 1989; 107:218–228.

40. Shami MJ, Freeman W, Friedberg D, et al. A multicenter study of *Pneumocystis* choroidopathy. Am J Ophthalmol 1991; 112:15–22.

41. Remington JS. Toxoplasmoss in the adult. Bull N Y Acad Med 1974; 50:211–227.

42. Glasner PD, Silveira C, Kruszon-Moran D, et al. An unusually high prevalence of ocular toxoplasmosis in southern Brazil. Am J Ophthalmol 1992; 114:136–144.

43. Soheilian M, Sadoughi MM, Ghajarnia M, et al. Prospective randomized trial of trimethoprim/sulfamethoxazole versus pyrimethamine and sulfadiazine in the treatment of ocular toxoplasmosis. Ophthalmology 2005; 112:1876–1882.

44. Silveira C, Belfort R Jr., Muccioli C, et al. The effect of long-term intermittent trimethoprim/sulfamethoxazole treatment on recurrences of toxoplasmic retinochoroiditis. Am J Ophthalmol 2002; 134:41–46.

45. Okada AA, Foster CS. Posterior uveitis in the pediatric population. Int Ophthalmol Clin 1992; 32:121–152.

46. Kotake S, Furudate N, Sasamoto Y, et al. Characteristics of endogenous uveitis in Hokkaido, Japan. Graefes Arch Clin Exp Ophthalmol 1997; 235:5–9.

47. Pivetti-Pezzi P, Accorinti M, La Cava M, et al. Endogenous uveitis: an analysis of 1,417 cases. Ophthalmologica 1996; 210:234–238.

48. International Study Group for Behçet's Disease. Criteria for diagnosis of Behçet's disease. Lancet 1990; 335:1078–1080.

49. Okada AA. Behçet's disease: general concepts and recent advances. Curr Opin Ophthalmol 2006; 17:551–556.

50. Kotter I, Zierhut M, Eckstein AK, et al. Human recombinant interferon alfa-2a for the treatment of Behçet's disease with sight threatening posterior or panuveitis. Br J Ophthalmol 2003; 87:423–431.

51. Ohno S, Nakamura S, Hori S, et al. Efficacy, safety and pharmacokinetics of multiple administration of infliximab in Behçet's disease with refractory uveoretinitis. J Rheumatol 2004; 31:1362–1368.

52. Atmaca LS, Batioglu F, Idil A. Retinal and disc neovascularization in Behçet's disease and efficacy of laser photocoagulation. Graefes Arch Clin Exp Ophthalmol 1996; 234:94–99.

53. Mitchell IC, Turk JL, Mitchell DN. Detection of mycobacterial rRNA in sarcoidosis with liquid-phase hybridization. Lancet 1992; 339:1015–1017.

54. Ishige I, Usui Y, Takemura T, et al. Quantitative PCR of mycobacterial and propionibacterial DNA in lymph nodes of Japanese patients with sarcoidosis. Lancet 1999; 354:120–123.

55. Kurokawa T, Kikuchi T, Ohta K, et al. Ocular manifestations in Blau syndrome associated with a CARD15/Nod2 mutation. Ophthalmology 2003; 110:2040–2044.

56. Read RW, Holland GN, Rao NA, et al. Revised diagnostic criteria for Vogt-Koyanagi-Harada disease: report of an international committee on nomenclature. Am J Ophthalmol 2001; 131:647–652.

57. Read RW, Rechodouni A, Butani N, et al. Complications and prognostic factors in Vogt-Koyanagi-Harada disease. Am J Ophthalmol 2001; 131:599–606.

58. Read RW, Yu F, Accorinti M, et al. Evaluation of the effect on outcomes of the route of administration of corticosteroids in acute and subacute Vogt-Koyanagi-Harada disease. Am J Ophthalmol 2006; 141:119–124.

59. Yamaki K, Hara K, Sakuragi S. Application of the revised diagnostic crtieria for Vogt-Koyanagi-Harada disease in Japanese patients. Jpn J Ophthalmol 2005; 49:143–148.

60. Okada AA, Mizusawa T, Sakai J, Usui M. Videofunduscopy and videoangiography using the scanning laser ophthalmoscope in patients with Vogt-Koyanagi-Harada syndrome. Br J Ophthalmol 1998; 82:1175–1181.

61. Kilmartin DJ, Dick AD, Forrester JV. Prospective surveillance of sympathetic ophthalmia in the United Kingdom and Republic of Ireland. Br J Ophthalmol 2000; 84:259–263.

62. Kilmartin DJ, Wilson D, Liversidge J, et al. Immunogenetic and clinical phenotype of sympathetic ophthalmia in British and Irish patients. Br J Ophthalmol 2001; 85:281–286.

63. Lightman S, McDonald WI, Bird AC, et al. Retinal venous sheathing in optic neuritis; its significance for the pathogenesis of multiple sclerosis. Brain 1987; 110:405–414.

64. Geier SA, Nasemann J, Klauss V, et al. Frosted branch angiitis associated with cytomegalovirus retinitis. Am J Ophthalmol 1992; 114:514–516.

65. Callanan D, Gass JDM. Multifocal choroiditis and choroidal neovascularization associated with the multiple evanescent white dot and acute idiopathic blind spot enlargement syndrome. Ophthalmology 1992; 99:1678–1685.

66. Tang J, Stevens RA, Okada AA, et al. Association of antiretinal antibodies in acute annular outer retinopathy. Arch Ophthalmol 2008; 126:130–132.

67. Watzke RC, Shults WT. Clinical features and natural history of the acute idiopathic enlarged blind spot syndrome. Ophthlamology 2002; 109:1326–1335.

68. Gass JDM. Acute zonal occult outer retinopathy. J Clin Neuroopthalmol 1993; 13:79–97.

69. Fekrat S, Wilkinson CP, Chang B, et al. Acute annular outer retinopathy: report of four cases. Am J Ophthalmol 2000; 130:636–644.

70. Wright BE, Bird AC, Hamilton AM. Placoid pigment epitheliopathy and Harada's disease. Br J Ophthalmol 1978; 62:609–621.

71. Akpek EK, Jabs DA, Tessler HH, et al. Successful treatment of serpiginous choroiditis with alkylating agents. Ophthalmology 2002; 109:1506–1513.

72. Jones BE, Jampol LM, Yannuzzi LA, et al. Relentless placoid chorioretinitis: a new entity or an unusual variant of serpiginous choroidopathy? Arch Ophthalmol 2000; 118:931–938.

73. Holland GN, Shah KH, Monnet D, et al. Longitudinal cohort study of patients with birdshot chorioretinopathy II: color vision at baseline. Am J Ophthalmol 2006; 142:1013–1018.

74. Monnet D, Brezin AP, Holland GN, et al. Longitudinal cohort study of patients withh birdshot chorioretinopathy I: baseline clinical characteristics. Am J Ophthalmol 2006; 141:135–142.

75. Holder GE, Robson AG, Pavesio C, Graham EM. Electrophysiological characterisation and monitoring in the management of birdshot chorioretinopathy. Br J Ophthalmol 2005; 89:709–718.

76. Levinson RD, Brezin A, Rothova A, et al. Research criteria for the diagnosis of birdshot chorioretinopathy: results of an international consensus conference. Am J Ophthalmol 2006; 141:185–187.

77. Nussenblatt RB, Palestine AG, Chan CC, et al. Standardization of vitreal inflammatory activity in intermediate and posterior uveitis. Ophthalmology 1985; 92:467–471.

78. Kiss S, Ahmed M, Letko E, et al. Long-term follow-up of patients with birdshot retinochoroidopathy treated with corticosteroid-sparing systemic immunomodulatory therapy. Ophthalmology 2005; 112:1066–1071.

79. Priem HA, Oosterhuis JA. Birdshot chorioretinopathy: clinical characteristics and evolution. Br J Ophthalmol 1988; 72:646–659.

80. Sobrin L, Lam BL, Liu M, et al. Electroretinographic monitoring in birdshot chorioretinopathy. Am J Ophthalmol 2005; 140:52–64.

81. Thorne JE, Wittenberg S, Jabs DA, et al. Multifocal choroiditis with panuveitis incidence of ocular complications and of loss of visual acuity. Ophthalmology 2006; 113:2310–2316.

82. Brown J, Folk JC, Reddy CV, et al. Visual prognosis of multifocal choroiditis, punctate inner choroidopathy, and the diffuse subretinal fibrosis syndrome. Ophthalmology 1996; 103:1100–1105.

83. Rothova A, Buitenhuis HJ, Meenken C, et al. Uveitis and systemic disease. Br J Ophthalmol 1992; 76:137–141.

84. Raja SC, Jabs DA, Dunn JP, et al. Pars planitis: clinical features and class II HLA associations. Ophthalmology 1999; 106:594–599.

85. Whitcup SM, Stark-Vancs V, Wittes RE, et al. Association of interleukin 10 in the vitreous and cerebrospinal fluid and primary central nervous system lymphoma. Arch Ophthalmol 1997; 115:1157–1160.

86. Davis JL. Diagnosis of intraocular lymphoma. Ocular Immunol Inflamm 2004; 12:7–16.

87. Smith JR, Rosenbaum JT, Wilson DJ, et al. Role of intravitreal methotrexate in the management of primary central nervous system lymphoma with ocular involvement. Ophthalmology 2002; 109:1709–1716.

4

Instituting and Monitoring Therapy for Sight-Threatening Uveitis

INTRODUCTION

Uveitis and indeed ocular inflammation generally present an unsettling challenge to the ophthalmologist for many reasons: first, the precise diagnosis of the inflammatory condition may not be obvious, and thus, the natural outcome of the disease may be unpredictable, which makes informed discussion with the patient difficult; second, even if the diagnosis is clear, the best treatment options may not be obvious, and the risks of treatment may be even less clear; third, even if the optimal treatment regime for any given patient is evident, most ophthalmologists are uneasy with the use of modern powerful immunosuppressants, which constitute the pharmacopoeia for controlling ocular inflammation, and thus, they usually rely on their physician colleagues to institute and monitor therapy; fourth, best practice for monitoring treatment is frequently an area of uncertainty since treatment protocols often have to be tailored to the patient's condition; finally, even if all the best advices are available from an expert in management of sight-threatening ocular inflammation (STOI), the cost of the treatment may be prohibitive even in developed countries with well funded health services.

In spite of the above stated challenges and uncertainties, the management of STOI is in fact quite straightforward. This chapter describes a simple, direct approach to the institution and particularly to the monitoring of STOI. The details of the specific immunosuppressants, both medical and surgical, are dealt with in chapter 5.

THE DECISION TO TREAT SIGHT THREATENING OCULAR INFLAMMATION (STOI)

The previous chapters have introduced and broadly overviewed "treating the patient presenting to the clinic/office with ocular inflammation" as well as detailing the many different types of intraocular inflammatory conditions and syndromes, and highlighting the various investigations that are helpful in reaching these diagnoses. However, the central purpose of performing investigations is to identify treatable causes of disease and, while a precise diagnosis can be very valuable in offering prognosis and predicting the outcome of disease, as highlighted in earlier chapters, it is not essential to the treatment of, or prevention of, irreversible visual loss from ocular inflammation. Once the clinical symptoms and signs have been definitively attributed to a primary ocular inflammation (and not some other cause such as masquerade syndrome or inflammation secondary to some other primary ocular disease such as undetected rhegmatogenous retinal detachment), the two main determinants of the type of treatment are

- whether the disease is infectious or noninfectious
- whether the inflammation is sight-threatening

This chapter focuses on the management of *sight-threatening disease.*

Treatment of Posterior Segment STOI

In chapter 2, we highlighted the features that identify STOI. However, it is important to emphasize that while sight-threatening posterior segment inflammation generally varies with the degree of inflammation, the correlation is not strong. For instance, some patients with considerable vitreous opacities due to previously active intermediate uveitis may experience significant intermittent interference in vision through the central visual axis, but their sight is not fundamentally under threat. Conversely, patients with conditions such as serpiginous choroidopathy in which the lesion is encroaching toward the fovea are under considerable visual threat and require urgent initiation of treatment. Simply determining a composite severity assessment clinically (chaps. 1 and 2) can assist in determining which treatment to institute (Box 1).

In most cases, the preferred treatment is systemic immunosuppression (1,2), although some ophthalmologists advocate periocular or even intravitreal administration of corticosteroids for mild and moderate cases, particularly if unilateral. There is evidence that local treatment is useful in control of mild to moderate intraocular inflammation, although it does require frequent ongoing administration (3,4). However, the rationale for local treatment is not clear since locally administered corticosteroids are less sensitive to regulated control than a daily administered systemic drug. In addition, a considerable proportion of the periocular

---

Box 1

In posterior segment intraocular inflammation (PSII), classify the level of severity of the threat to vision as

Minimal: No treatment necessary

Mild: Treatment may be necessary (local periocular or systemic corticosteroid)

Moderate: Treatment required [corticosteroid (tapering dose from 0.5 mg/kg) $\pm$ second-line immunosuppression]

Severe: Urgent, aggressive treatment required (see below)

---

drug is adsorbed systemically (similar to an intramuscular injection), and it is likely that a considerable part of its effect is mediated through the systemic route. The risk of undertreatment with this approach is considerable since the ophthalmologist falls into a false sense of security that there is a prolonged depot effect, while, in fact, there is an exponential decline in the effective concentration of drug (5–7).

Treatment of Anterior Segment STOI

Sight-threatening anterior segment ocular inflammation is much less common (Box 2). Most cases do not represent a direct threat to sight provided the potential secondary complications of untreated inflammation such as pupillary seclusion, cataract, and glaucoma are controlled with topical steroid and cycloplegic therapies.

Most cases also do not require prolonged systemic therapy, and a short course of systemic corticosteroids is often sufficient to control the inflammation.

Box 2

In anterior segment disease, the threat to sight can be categorized as

Minimal: Only topical treatment required

Mild: Only Topical treatment required

Moderate: Systemic treatment if not controlled (short course of corticosteroids)

Severe: Systemic treatment usually required (see below)

However, continuing inflammation may require a second-line drug such as methotrexate, cyclosporine, tacrolimus, or mycophenolate mofetil, which can be tapered after a few weeks of stabilization (8–10). It is well recognized that preventing anterior segment STOI may require prolonged chronic use in childhood in JIA-associated uveitis to prevent blindness in adulthood. The ocular complications of JIA-associated uveitis are high compared to other forms of anterior uveitis: the incidence of bilateral disease is between 67% and 85%, and complications of uveitis are reported in 20% to 40% of children at presentation and steadily accumulate over the first two decades of life, especially in those with persistently active disease. The result, despite current immunosuppression, is that 10% end up being visually impaired.

AIMS OF TREATMENT

It is essential in any treatment protocol for the physician to have a clear idea of the aims of his treatment and to present these simply and logically to his patient with full information on risk and benefits of the therapy. It is then the duty of the treating physician to offer the patient the best advice he can for the patient's individual care based on current knowledge and to obtain informed consent from the patient before initiating therapy.

In the initial stages of the disease, the primary aim is to remove the *immediate* threat to sight, and for this purpose, corticosteroids are the most effective agents if used at high-enough doses and have a fast onset of significant immunosuppression. In many cases, even when the signs are not florid, as in patients with uveitis-associated cystoid macular edema, a short sharp course of intravenous methylprednisolone can have a dramatic effect on both visual acuity and objective signs of macular edema (chap. 2, page 46). The only major caveat to early institution of steroid therapy is that in certain cases of infectious STOI, there is a risk of worsening the condition (see below).

Once the threat to sight has been removed, it is important to *sustain* the clinical improvement by instituting the second-line drugs, if possible simultaneously. This is in part because of the fact that some of these drugs such as cyclosporine and tacrolimus take some days to achieve therapeutic effect when delivered orally since they are stored in body fats, and methotrexate and antimetabolites have a much prolonged onset of significant immunosuppressive action. Irrespective of the choice of immunosuppressant (chap. 5), it is essential to perform baseline laboratory investigations to exclude pretreatment systemic morbidity, which may be exacerbated by toxic effects of immunosuppression, and to use these baseline readings to monitor changes that may occur as a result of drug toxicity.

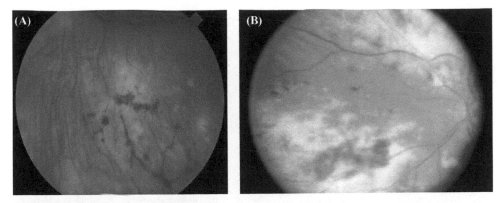

Figure 1 Spectrum of herpetic retinopathy presenting as sight-threatening ocular inflammation. (**A**) demonstrates the cardinal features of early acute retinal necrosis with vasculitis, hemorrhage, and early retinal edema and necrosis as a result of herpes simplex. (**B**) demonstrates a more florid retinitis (secondary to CMV) in an immunocompromised patient.

Infectious Posterior Segment STOI

As indicated above, in cases where infection is the major threat to sight, treatment of the infection is paramount. In such cases, diagnosis is important, and fortunately, many infectious causes of STOI are recognizable by their clinical signs. This includes viral diseases such as CMV retinitis or Herpes viridae-associated acute retinal necrosis (Fig. 1) in which steroid therapy is contra-indicated because of the risk of worsening the condition.

Some causes of infectious uveitis are, however, benefited from the early introduction of corticosteroids since this minimizes collateral damage induced by the innate immune response to the dead and dying organisms. In the case of toxoplasmosis, there is not as yet universal agreement on the use corticosteroids, and in some cases the use of corticosteroids before institution of specific therapy can risk visual loss (Fig. 2). In practice, the careful and timely introduction of corticosteroids in sight-threatening toxoplasmosis has a beneficial effect.

In many cases, the diagnosis of infectious STOI is difficult and a heightened sense of awareness is the best diagnostic aid. For instance, miliary tuberculosis presents in many ways as, for example, one of the white dot syndromes [e.g., multiple evanescent white dot syndrome (MEWDS)] (Fig. 3) and may not be associated with significant visual loss, in the early stages. A high index of suspicion, however, allows diagnostic confirmation (in this case via renal biopsy and specific culture). In TB-associated STOI, specific therapy combined with immunosuppression is the correct management. In fact, the dose of systemic corticosteroids in active tuberculosis is twice the standard therapy (chap. 5) since there is considerable suppression of steroid metabolism as a result of enzyme induction from rifampicin.

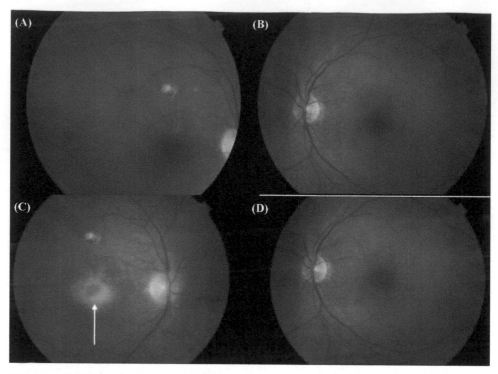

Figure 2 Development of toxoplasmosis following immunosuppression for presumed non-infectious PSII. (**A**, **B**) show patient presenting with early features of PSII and treated with steroids. (**C**, **D**) show development of toxoplasma choroiditis (*arrow*) following immunosuppression. *Abbreviation*: PSII, posterior segment intraocular inflammation.

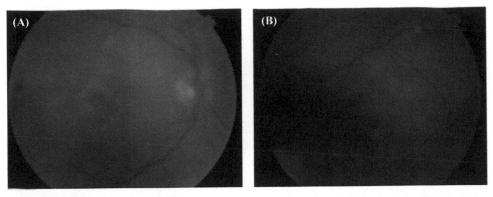

Figure 3 Miliary tuberculosis presenting as a white dot syndrome. A, B show multifocal chorioretinal lesions centrally and peripherally, respectively.

Difficulties arise in cases of multiple infections, for example, combined toxoplasmosis and herpesvirus retinitis in immunocompromised patients or indeed infection as a result of immunosuppression in inflammatory disease or cases of low-grade chronic endophthalmitis in postsurgical patients. In the latter case, the typical clinical course is of a good response to moderate-dose steroid therapy with a less good response to additional immunosuppression, and recurrence when the drugs are tapered. Continuing low-grade vitritis with cystoid macular edema leads to progressive macular damage. Clinical awareness and diagnostic vitrectomy (with culture, sensitivity, and PCR testing) help to provide accurate diagnosis and an appropriate treatment plan. Where immunosuppression is indicated, the institution of therapy should be along the lines of noninfectious posterior segment STOI as detailed below (Box 3).

Box 3
Where infectious posterior segment STOI is diagnosed or strongly suspected specific treatment should be guided by blood and ocular fluid culture/PCR studies and instituted as a generic guide as follows:

Bacterial endophthalmitis: Intravitreal and systemic antibiotics
CMV: Systemic ganciclovir, or valganciclovir
VZV/HSV: Acyclovir or equivalent
(In viral retinitis local intraocular treatments may be warranted—foscarnet, ganciclovir implant)
Fungal: Intravitreal and systemic antifungals

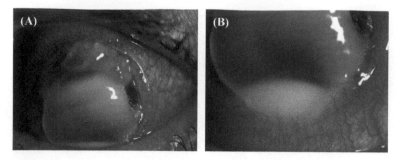

Figure 4 Infectious keratitis and corneal melt. In this patient, there is a severe corneal/peripheral ulcerative keratitis melt (**A**), which has led to corneal edema and anterior segment sight-threatening ocular inflammation, with intraocular infection and hypopyon (**B**).

Infectious Anterior Segment STOI

The same principles apply to the institution of therapy in infectious anterior segment STOI. Many cases of infectious keratouveitis/endophthalmitis are clinically obvious (Fig. 4), for instance, by the presence of an infected corneal ulcer (e.g., in contact lens wearers) or surgical wound (e.g., "blebitis," which is becoming more common because of the use of antimetabolites in glaucoma surgery). In these cases, concurrent systemic immunosuppression is rarely required, and appropriate topical and systemic antibiotic therapy, guided by microbiological studies for organism culture and sensitivity, is the correct management. In the responding stages of the condition, judicious use of topical corticosteroids may minimize tissue damage and promote healing.

More difficult to recognize are the cases of anterior segment infectious STOI where an infectious agent is not immediately detectable [e.g., in Posner-Schlossman sydnrome or glaucomatocyclitic crisis, a condition with self-limited recurrent episodes of markedly elevated intraocular pressure (IOP) with mild idiopathic anterior chamber inflammation]. Many cases of unilateral, recurrent anterior uveitis are caused by HSV (Fig. 5) (or indeed others of the herpes family), which responds partially to topical corticosteroids but recur with a vengeance on tapering the drugs, often in conjunction with secondary glaucoma and corneal edema. It is then difficult to differentiate between infectious keratouveitis, steroid-induced glaucoma, and glaucoma secondary to the ocular inflammation. Meanwhile, there is a significant reduction in vision, which may become irretrievable as the corneal opacification persists and becomes permanent.

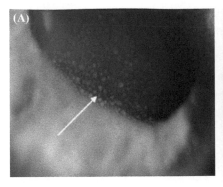 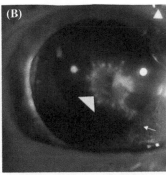

Figure 5 Anterior segment signs of herpetic anterior uveitis. (**A**) displays keratic precipitates (*arrow*). (**B**) shows localized cataract from previous posterior synaechia and seclusio pupillae (*arrowhead*) and iris atrophy (*arrow*).

In such cases, it may be useful to stop all treatment (apart from the antiglaucoma therapy) and to institute a course of systemic antiviral therapy such as acyclovir at high doses (400–800 mg five times daily) for several weeks. A helpful diagnostic sign in such cases is sectoral iris atrophy or evidence of iris pigment epithelial dropout, and the exclusive unilaterality of the disease frequently permits differentiation from noninfectious anterior uveitis, which is frequently bilateral, or in the case of HLA B27-associated anterior uveitis, alternating between eyes. In addition, PCR testing for virus can be especially useful if positive.

Noninfectious Posterior Segment STOI

Instituting Systemic Steroid Therapy

As indicated above, once infection has been excluded from the diagnosis, rapid introduction of corticosteroid therapy is required to control inflammation and prevent permanent visual loss. This is particularly so where the threat to vision is judged to be severe (see above). This may require high-dose intravenous methylprednisolone (1 g once daily for three days in adults), and should be instituted even where, as we indicated in the introduction, there is considerable disparity between the threat to sight and the clinical signs of inflammation, necessitating strong and rapid immunosuppression. To emphasize this point, one of the main sites of visual threat is the fovea and cases in which there is significant cystoid edema, where there is a leaking inflammatory choroidal neovascular membrane (CNV) (Fig. 6) or where there is encroachment of a serpiginous tongue into the juxtafoveal region (Fig. 7), intravenous corticosteroids

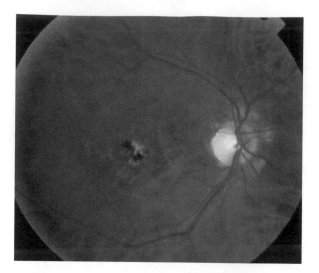

Figure 6   Fundus color photograph of inflammatory choroidal neovascular membrane.

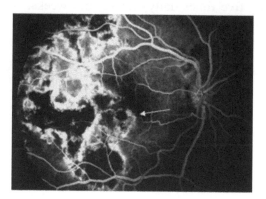

Figure 7   Fundus fluorescein angiogram of posterior segment sight-threatening ocular inflammation. Arrow shows the sight-threatening extension of serpiginous lesion toward the fovea.

will rapidly halt this progression and buy time for the introduction of additional therapies.

Second-line therapies include cyclosporine A, tacrolimus, mycophenolate mofetil, methotrexate, and azathioprine (8–11). The choice drug is determined by the general health status of the patient including assessment of hematological, renal, and biochemical parameters, and also where evidence exists for their efficacy (chap. 5).

Box 4
Severe Disease

Following intravenous corticosteroids, a rapidly tapering dose of oral corticosteroids should be introduced customized to the health and visual needs of the patients.

60 mg prednisolone for three days
40 mg prednisolone for one week
30 mg prednisolone for one or two weeks
20 mg for one to three weeks, depending on the severity of disease and the associated side effects.

Then gradual reduction of the steroid dose either to 15 mg daily followed by weekly 1 mg dose reduction to a baseline dose of 10 mg or even slower reduction, not unusually by 1 mg every two weeks or even by 1 mg monthly, depending on the risk of reactivation (There are no hard and fast rules, as consensus has not been set, except that relapse occurs often when the corticosteroids are reduced too rapidly.)

Some patients with less severe or *moderate* threat to sight may not require initial treatment with intravenous methylprednisolone, but will respond to a moderate to high dose of oral corticosteroids, for example, prednisolone @ 0.75 to 1 mg/kg/day. This can be continued for three to five days, and the tapering plan outlined as per *severe* disease (Box 4) can be instituted. It is important to emphasize that fine-tuning this regime in response to the patient's needs both from the improvement-in-vision response and the development of side effects is the best way to customize this treatment protocol for each individual.

Patients with *mild* threat to sight may not need oral corticosteroids as initial therapy but will require supervision and possibly some form of immunosuppression to reduce their risk of gradual visual loss. Some advocate use of local depot corticosteroids as per orbital floor, subtenon's, or intraocular injections. While there is evidence for efficacy (3,4), there is also a requirement for long-term repeated treatments. Others advocate that these patients can be introduced directly to the "second-line" drugs (chap. 5), and in such cases, low-dose tacrolimus or mycophenolate mofetil may be very useful to maintain longer-term control, particularly in bilateral cases.

Instituting "Second-Line" Immunosuppression

The aim of treatment is to maintain visual improvement on the lowest effective and tolerable dose of immunosuppression as possible (8,9). Since corticosteroids have such a wide range of side effects (see below), a primary aim is to try to reduce the dose of corticosteroids to zero, or at least to less than 10 mg daily (preferably <7.5 mg daily). This is one of the reasons why treatment devolves to the use of other drugs. A second reason is that "second-line" immunosuppression offers additional therapeutic benefits (Box 5). Although anecdotally there is a strong view for single treatment with second-line agents, there remains little evidence to date. However, recent studies with long-term mycophenolate mofetil (10) and tacrolimus (11) use show that there is about an 80% to 85% probability of reducing corticosteroid dose to below 10 mg in one year of treatment.

In the early days of steroid control of uveitis, azathioprine and methotrexate (12) were recommended and more commonly used as "steroid-sparing" drugs. Particularly with methotrexate, this remains well tolerated and has superior "retention time" to many other immunosuppressives (13). However, experience (no direct head-to-head trial data) has taught that these drugs in isolation are arguably less effective in preventing recurrences of uveitis and eventual visual loss. Other drugs such as chlorambucil are rarely used because of their considerable side effects and overall inferior efficacy.

As indicated above, it is important to institute therapy with one of these agents in tandem with inflammation-controlling steroid therapy since once the

---

Box 5
Second Line Immunosuppressives

- *Cyclosporin* has now been used as a major therapeutic agent for control of uveitis (1) and has been shown to be very effective. It is currently used at a loading dose of 5 mg/kg body weight and tapered to a minimal effective dose over several weeks, with maintenance at 2.5 mg/kg/day.
- *Tacrolimus* (FK506) has been shown to be equally effective with an improved quality of life (less perceived side effects)(2) and currently this is the preferred management (initiating dose 1–2 mg daily and titrated to serum levels of 5–9 ng/mL).
- *Mycophenolate mofetil* has more recently been shown to be effective in control of mild to moderate sight-threatening uveitis (initial dose 500 mg b.i.d. and increased to maintenance of 1 g b.i.d.) (10).

corticosteroids are tapered, the likelihood of disease recrudescence is strong, particularly in moderate to severe disease (8).

In summary, many patients can have their STOI controlled on a low dose of prednisolone (<10 mg daily) with a second-line agent, and, as indicated above, the aim of therapy is to reduce the requirement for both drugs either to monotherapy usually with the second-line agent, or to no therapy. Reaching this desired goal can take several weeks to months but in some cases is achievable, particularly in patients with inflammatory CNVs (chap. 5). Recrudescences may occur in the form of visual distortion from extension of the membrane and in these cases, the above treatment protocol may have to be resumed, beginning with the intravenous methylprednisolone particularly in one-eyed patients with or without associated photodynamic therapy (PDT) or anti-VEGF (Vascular Endothelial Growth Factor) therapies.

However, in some patients, complete tapering of their drug therapy is not possible, and in these cases it is important to achieve the lowest effective therapeutic dose of either drug or both drugs in combination (see next section). Some of these patients may be on therapy for a very long period (years) with increasing risk of life-threatening side effects such as tumor, cardiovascular disease, or renal failure, thus the need for full informed consent.

Combination Therapy

Combination therapy is the *norm* rather than the exception in treatment of posterior segment STOI and has increasing popularity (8,9). Usually, this is a low-dose steroid combined with a calcineurin inhibitor (cyclosporine or tacrolimus) or an antimetabolite (mycophenolate mofetil, azathioprine, methotrexate). However, the threat to sight may be difficult to control with low-dose therapy, and/or an increase in either of the two mainstay drugs may be accompanied with unacceptable side effects. In such circumstances, it is appropriate to consider adding a third [and very occasionally even a fourth drug to achieve good control, although now most would use *biologic therapy for maintained drug-induced remission* (chap. 5)] while minimizing the side effects of each drug. Thus, a significant threat of visual loss in a patient may be controlled with a combination of low-dose prednisolone (<10 mg daily), tacrolimus (2 mg twice daily), and mycophenolate mofetil (1 g twice daily).

Clearly, this is a risky strategy, and close monitoring of the patient is essential. If control is not achieved using this strategy or if side effects become unacceptable, consideration of one of the newer "biologics" may be the next step (chap. 5). This may require a drug washout period (in the case of interferon therapy) since immunosuppression may interfere with the action of the biologic, and in such cases, very careful adjustment of therapy is required to avoid irreversible visual loss [e.g., from vascular occlusion in Behcet's retinal vasculitis (chap. 3)].

Use of Local Corticosteroids

In less severe cases and in particular in unilateral cases of moderate STOI with macular edema, many ophthalmologists advocate the use of local (periocular, "orbital floor," subconjunctival) corticosteroids to control the inflammation, repeated at intervals depending on whether the disease recurs and vision deteriorates. Intravitreal corticosteroids are also used by some (intravitreal triamcinolone, long acting steroid intravitreal inserts) particularly where the risk of side effects is too great.

The main difficulty with local corticosteroids is that drug delivery is erratic and not controlled, whereas intravenous and oral corticosteroids can be regulated very rapidly by withholding or increasing the drug dose. In addition, studies have shown that there is a considerable systemic absorption particularly of periocular injections, and that in fact the most effective periocular route in achieving high premacular concentrations of corticosteroids is subconjuctival (5). Thus, the rationale for periocular injections is not strong.

The disadvantage of intravitreal steroid injections or steroid-releasing implants is the high incidence of complications, particularly cataract and glaucoma, with a lesser but real risk of retinal detachment and endophthalmitis. Local and intravitreal drug administration for STOI is also available only for corticosteroids, thus restricting its use to mild or more moderate cases of STOI.

Noninfectious Anterior Segment STOI

Instituting Steroid Therapy All cases of active anterior segment STOI should be treated with topical corticosteroids provided infectious causes have been ruled out. In addition, cycloplegics are almost always required to prevent posterior synechiae and seclusion of the pupil. Topical therapy should be continued until such time as the inflammation has resolved. Raised IOP should also be managed with appropriate antiglaucoma therapy (chap. 5).

Some cases of anterior segment STOI fail to respond to such therapy even if intensively applied. In such cases, periocular (subconjunctival) corticosteroids are extremely effective (see below). Suspicion of posterior segment disease should be raised if there is a poor view of the fundus and vision loss appears out of proportion to the level of inflammation. Even if posterior segment disease is discounted (e.g., by echography), consideration of systemic steroid therapy may be necessary. In such cases, oral corticosteroids are usually sufficient (protocol as for *moderate* posterior segment STOI discussed above).

Instituting second-line immunosuppression Rarely, prolonged use of oral corticosteroids is unable to control anterior segment STOI and second-line immunosuppression is required, for instance in conditions where longer-term control is required following inadequate control with topical and systemic steroids [such as, JIA-associated uveitis (14)]. In such cases, the protocols as for posterior segment disease are appropriate. Prolonged treatment in STOI restricted to the anterior segment is rarely necessary, and the condition settles after a few weeks. Thus, drug tapering here is much more rapid and manageable. However, topical therapy may have to be continued for some time after cessation of systemic therapy.

Combination therapy It is very rare that two or more drugs are required for control of anterior segment STOI [apart from JIA-associated uveitis in children; biologics may have to be prescribed in some of these cases (14)]. However, there are certain conditions of anterior segment inflammation that are considered by the ophthalmologists to be selectively "surface disease" and not intraocular: these are the atopic/allergic keratitic disorders, often associated with severe but not recognized atopic skin disease. Such patients respond moderately to systemic steroid therapy but frequently develop steroid toxicity; however, they respond well to second-line immunosuppressants, particularly cyclosporine, tacrolimus, and mycophenolate mofetil. In addition, the skin disease coincidentally often responds very well, and overall, their general well-being improves. Treatment may have to be prolonged for months to years but can be controlled with very low doses. It is important to remember the risk of carcinoma, especially carcinoma-in-situ in these cases.

Use of local corticosteroids As indicated above, topical steroid therapy is a sine qua non in anterior segment inflammation. Subconjuctival injections for severe fibrinous anterior uveitis are very effective and may be repeated within 24 hours. Subconjunctival mydriatics are also very valuable in breaking developing synechiae. Orbital floor and peribulbar corticosteroids are not indicated here, nor are intravitreal injections/implants.

INVESTIGATION PRIOR TO TREATMENT

There are two main reasons for undertaking investigations in patients with STOI, which are

- to make a diagnosis and
- to evaluate the patient's state of health prior to instituting treatment.

This section deals with investigations prior to treatment.

Box 6
A range of laboratory investigations are required.

- Hematology: Including hemtocrit and blood film
- Biochemistry: Including electrolyte measurements and liver function tests
- Radiology: Chest X ray (CXR) plus other imaging as indicated by clinical examination
- Renal Function: Blood urea nitrogen (BUN), serum creatinine, estimated GFR (eGFR)
- Immunology: erythrocyte sedimentation rate (ESR), other acute phase reactants—plasma viscosity, C-reactive protein; protein electrophoresis
- Urinalysis: Glucose, proteinuria

Noninfectious uveitis can be regarded as an organ-specific systemic disease presenting in the eye, similar to other organ-specific diseases such as thyroiditis or diabetes mellitus. The consequences are equally life-threatening (blindness!). Therefore, a full medical investigation is required, beginning with a documented systematic history and clinical examination to elicit symptoms and signs of associated disease. In many cases of uveitis, however, they may prove negative, which gives us important information in its own right.

In addition, it is important to exclude pregnancy or the risk of pregnancy in women of child-bearing age. Notwithstanding other investigations that may be driven by clinical examination (chaps. 2 and 3), baseline investigations for safety and monitoring of immunosuppression are required (see Box 6 for outline of investigations required).

Infectious STOI

Certain clinical and laboratory studies will help to exclude infectious uveitis: these include general examination, in particular checking for fever, lymphadenopathy, history of previous infections, for example, gastrointestinal or genitor-urinary tract infections and similar medical tests. In general, routine testing is not indicated, but urine, stool, blood, and cerebral spinal fluid (CSF) cultures and PCR studies should all be performed as and if indicated.

Noninfectious STOI

Since most of the immunosuppressants affect several of the body's organ systems, it is useful to include a checklist of organ function before instituting therapy (Box 7).

Box 7

- Corticosteroids: Random glucose, glucose, bone density, psychometrics, skin disease
- Calcineurin inhibitors: Renal, liver, and hematological blood tests Inquire about history of previous tumors especially in replicating sites such as skin and bone marrow.
- Antimetabolites: Hematological and liver function tests and systems inquiry regarding gastrointestinal tract and anemia[1]

---

[1]For azathioprine enzyme testing, *Thiopurine methyltransferase* (TMPT) levels should be assayed to predict possible acute bone marrow suppression in low TMPT expressers. For methotrexate, exclude macrocytic anemia and folate deficiency.

MONITORING RESPONSE TO TREATMENT/ ASSESSING SEVERITY

As indicated above, the main aim of treatment is to control inflammation with the lowest effective dose of immunosuppression, and thus, all patients who are returning to the clinic for review, whose inflammation is stabilized, and who have achieved their best possible visual recovery should be evaluated actively for drug dose reduction. In the best example, this will lead to drug cessation without reactivation of disease. Monitoring of certain drugs is assisted by measuring trough levels of blood drug concentration (*tacrolimus and cyclosporine A*), for which regional laboratories have reference values. Following a period of drug-induced remission for 6 to 12 months, when the drug level is within the therapeutic reference range, reduce the drug dose further until after a further 3 to 6 months the drug can be stopped, unless reactivations occur, in which case judicious increases in the drug are necessary, followed, after restabilization of disease, by a further attempt to taper the drug dose, perhaps using smaller-dose reductions each time. The judgement of the treating ophthalmologists is important here, and experience is a great tutor.

Although monitoring the response to treatment follows a similar pattern in many clinics, the precise methods can show considerable variation from unit to unit. This has led to difficulties in comparing the results of different studies of the effects of new or even standard drug regimes. Accordingly, a standardized protocol for evaluating clinical symptoms and signs of uveitis has been devised by an international group of experts (the standardised uveitis nomenclature SUN guidelines), intended to introduce a simple and comparable approach to assessing intraocular inflammation (15). **It is**

recommended that this approach be adopted in routine practice and without question for use in published clinical trials.

    Monitoring drug efficacy is usually evaluated using the parameters detailed below (also chap. 2), where appropriate reference to the SUN guidelines is made. Monitoring drug safety is dealt with in a later section.

Vision

The most direct measure of drug efficacy is recovery and preservation of vision. Normally, this means visual acuity and is best evaluated using the early treatment diabetic retinopathy study (ETDRS) visual acuity chart for accurate and statistical grading of improvement. However, many units rely on standard Snellen acuity measurements.

    Measuring visual acuity alone, however, may be insufficient to assess the threat to vision. Many patients complain of visual distortion or haziness/loss of contrast, for instance, patients with CNV encroaching into the juxtafoveal area or with developing cystoid macular edema, and here measurement of contrast (using contrast gratings) or paracentral scotomata using the Amsler grid can be very sensitive to change.

    Some patients may have lost a considerable amount of central visual acuity but retain significant peripheral vision. Visual field assessment using both Goldmann fields and central visual fields are useful objective measures.

    Color vision evaluation can also sometimes be helpful particularly in optic nerve inflammation, and is best for assessing change, particularly a positive treatment response.

Clinical Ocular Examination

Although covered in previous chapters, in the context of instituting and monitoring therapy for STOI, it is worth reemphasizing here. Monitoring the response to treatment by clinical ocular examination involves assessing signs of *active* inflammation (Box 8); recording signs of previous inflammation such as posterior synechiae or healed chorioretinal scars, does not assist in evaluating the current disease state and whether the disease is coming under control. Differentiating between active and old/healed lesions can sometimes be difficult.

Ocular Investigations

Certain ocular investigations are very helpful in evaluating response to treatment. However, it is important to note that *not all* investigations will be helpful, and careful selection of the appropriate test will allow accurate assessment of activity

---

Box 8
Signs of active posterior segment disease
(Grading includes SUN recommendations)
Anterior segment:

- Flare/cells, iris vessel engorgement

Posterior segment:

- Vitreous haze {Binocular indirect ophthalmoscopy (BIO) grade[1]—a combination of both cells and protein exudate}
- Retinal vasculitis/vessel engorgement
- Edema (macular, optic nerve, subretinal, retinal detachment)
- Chorioretinal infiltrates (size and extent)
- Active chorioretinal lesions

---

[1]Vitreous cells can form aggregates and appear as snowballs (fig. 9) or in pars planitis as a "snowbank". However, this can be difficult to quantify, although a decrease in snowbank size can occur over time with appropriate treatment.

particularly if used sequentially for comparison in following disease progress. Many of the ancillary tests used to monitor disease have been introduced in chapter 2 (pg. 36–42). Selective tests are reiterated here to provide an overview when monitoring therapy.

Fundus Photography

This is a classical standard method for recording pathology in the fundus. More recently it has been used to produce standard photographs for evaluation of "vitreous haze" (BIO score) (16).

Fundus Fluorescein Angiography

Although not quantitative, fluorescein angiography (FA) is very sensitive in detecting signs of posterior segment STOI macular edema (leakage of dye in the macular area), vasculitis (leakage from vessels), and active CNV. In addition, detection of subtle chorioretinal infiltrates, which are hypofluorescent in early phases of the angiogram and hyperfluorescent in the later phases, can reveal considerably more activity than might be apparent on fundus examination.

Indocyanine Green Angiography

This can be useful in detecting activity in fundus lesions at a deeper level as in birdshot retinochoroidopathy (chap. 2) but is not usually very helpful for monitoring changes in activity.

Optical Coherence Tomography

Optical coherence tomography (OCT) has moved evaluation of retinal thickness and macular edema in particular onto a quantitative objective level, especially with the third generation and later version of the technology. Rapid changes in macular profiles can be seen in response to treatment, for instance, in response to systemic corticosteroids (Fig. 8) or IFNα. Faithful registration of images allows for sequential studies on the same eye, and numerical evaluation of retinal thickness has strong value in clinical trials. As for all methods of evaluating macular changes, correlation with visual function, especially visual acuity, is not absolute.

Electrophysiology

Some cases of severe visual loss due to STOI, such as advanced birdshot retinochoroidopathy and severe Behcet's retinal vasculitis with optic nerve atrophy, may still benefit from some low-level visual improvement or stabilization with immunosuppression. In such cases, the only objective measure of visual change may come from electrophysiological studies such as electroretinography and visual evoked potentials.

Ultrasonography

Imaging of the fundal periphery may be difficult, particularly in cases of panuveitis with extensive posterior synechiae or pars planitis with very peripheral chorioretinal

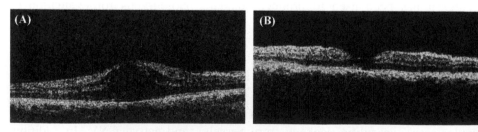

Figure 8 OCT images of a patient with steroid responsive CME. This patient with JIA-associated uveitis and CME. (**A**) shows a dramatic response to IV methylprednisolone therapy, after which the CME resolved by day 3 (**B**). *Abbreviation*: OCT, optical coherence tomography; CME, cystoid macular edema.

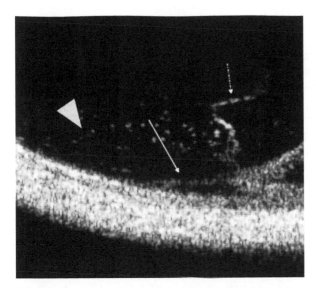

Figure 9 Ultrasound biomicroscopy (UBM). Snowballs and cellular aggregates can be visualized (*arrowhead*) at the pars plana and contraction of the vitreous base (*arrow*). Anterior hyaloid is clearly visible (*interrupted arrow*). UBM is useful for assessing disease in the pars plana, where the clinical view is restricted. It can facilitate understanding of peripheral vitreoretinal/ciliary body pathology and for decisions relating to appropriateness of vitreoretinal surgery.

deposits. In such cases, ultrasonography may be useful (Fig. 9) and evidence of reduction in deposits can be observed after prolonged treatment. Moreover, it allows assessment of vitreoretinal/ciliary body architecture, where the view is clinically difficult, and facilitates decision on surgical approaches and therapy.

MONITORING THE EMERGENCE OF SIDE EFFECTS

As indicated above, the dual role of the treating ophthalmologist is to monitor both the response to treatment and the side effects, and it is best if this is the same individual, that is, a medical ophthalmologist or ophthalmic physician trained in the management of ocular inflammation.

The number of immunosuppressive drugs is relatively limited, and with experience, the treating physician can gain expertise in early detection of side effects. This may involve the use of a symptom and sign checklist, which comprehensively covers the physiological and organ systems. Indeed, questionnaires are available and have been extensively used in quality of life studies that deal with such a set of questions (17,18). The systems that should be addressed directly with some examples of symptoms are detailed in Box 9.

Box 9

Gastrointestinal:	Nausea, diarrhea
Skin:	Rashes, pruritis
Neurological:	Dizziness, agitation
Musculoskeletal:	Cramps
Renal:	Lethary, lumbar pain
Hepatic:	Nausea, anorexia, lethargy, jaundice
Hematological:	Tiredness, fatigue
Biochemistry:	Cramps, dehydration
Metabolic:	Polyuria

These can be checked out, for instance, by the nurse practitioner at the clinic in a tick box fashion (Table 1).

Some drugs have well recognized side effects, which can be reduced by lowering the dose. For instance, mycophenolate mofetil is well-known to induce gastrointestinal disturbance at higher doses (diarrhea, nausea, and vomiting). Cyclosporine causes renal dysfunction in around 50% of patients even at low dose, manifested by a rise in serum creatinine and linked to hypertension. Tacrolimus causes less renal disturbance than cyclosporine but is more likely to cause liver dysfunction. Azathioprine can be involved in significant drug interactions and may rarely cause profound and difficult-to-reverse bone marrow aplasia.

Table 1 Check List for Adverse Drug Effects

System	Drug				
	Corticosteroids	Cyclosporin	Tacrolimus	Mycophenolate Mofetil	Azathioprine
GI tract					
GU tract					
Skin					
CNS					
Joints					
Renal					
Hepatic					
Haematol					
Biochemical					
Renal					
Metabolic					

Abbreviations: GI, gastrointestinal; GU, genitourinary; CNS, central nervous system.

Of all drugs commonly used, systemic corticosteroids have the strongest reputation for side effects. This includes mild to moderate psychosis, fluid retention, osteoporosis, moon facies and buffalo hump, hypertension, diabetes mellitus, acneiform rashes, and many other side effects. Overtreatment with corticosteroids is usually clinically obvious as the patient enters the clinic room and is so frequent that it has been the main reason for the development of newer therapies.

It is extremely important however to remember that the newer drugs have a quantifiable risk (around 3% overall) of tumor development, not directly as a result of the drugs but because of suppression of the immune response to cancer-inducing organisms (viruses). Thus, skin cancers and hematological tumors are the most common tumors and are linked to EB virus and papilloma virus exposure. This risk is not specific to any one drug, and is present even with prolonged steroid use. The risk increases with the duration of drug use and with increasing number of drugs used in combination. There have been a number of recent reviews of side effects of immunosuppression in treatment of uveitis (8,18).

Osteoporosis

For corticosteroids, it is important to gain risk factors and bone density measurements [dual-energy X-ray absorptiometry (DXA) scan] and incorporate regional/national guidelines for prophylaxis or treatment of osteoporosis. Osteoporosis may be defined as a disease with bone mineral density 2.5 or more standard deviations below normal peak bone mass (T score of −2.5 or less), but fragility fractures in patients taking corticosteroids appear to occur at a higher bone mineral density than in age-related or postmenopausal osteoporosis. Bone mineral density alone is therefore a poor predictor of fragility fractures in patients taking corticosteroids, and so it is important to also look at other risk factors for osteoporosis when deciding on treatment, including the body mass index (BMI), smoking, sex, age, and family history. For example (and there are subtle variances worldwide), the Royal College of Physicians (United Kingdom) has published guidelines on the prevention and treatment of glucocorticoid-induced osteoporosis. They recommend that

- the risk of osteoporosis is assessed in all patients who are committed to or have taken oral glucocorticoids for three or more months.
- patients aged 65 or more and patients who have had a previous fragility fracture or fracture while taking corticosteroids should be started on treatment as a preventative measure.
- all other patients should have their bone mineral density measured by a DXA scan and should be started on treatment if the T score is −1.5 or

lower. Alendronate, cyclic etidronate, and risedronate are licensed for the treatment of glucocorticoid-induced osteoporosis in United Kingdom.

- the American College of Rheumatology advises that all patients receive calcium and vitamin D supplementation and that bisphosphonates are prescribed in patients in whom the T score is below −1.

Monitoring of drug responses to biologic agents requires an approach similar to that described here but has certain additional requirements in regulating administration of drugs. These are described in chapter 5.

CONCLUSION

The management of STOI may at once appear difficult and dangerous, and less than effective in control of inflammation and preservation of vision. However, the approach to all drugs can be managed easily with the simple protocols outlined above, and many patients will preserve sight for prolonged periods and perhaps beyond the time when their disease will have been "burnt out". Management of these patients allows the art to be added back to the science of medical therapy.

REFERENCES

1. Dick AD, Azim M, Forrester JV. Immunosuppressive therapy for chronic uveitis: optimising therapy with steroids and cyclosporin A. Br J Ophthalmol 1997; 81(12): 1107–1112.
2. Murphy CC, Greiner K, Plskova J, et al. Cyclosporine vs tacrolimus therapy for posterior and intermediate uveitis. Arch Ophthalmol 2005; 123(5):634–641.
3. Antcliff RJ, Spalton DJ, Stanford MR, et al. Intravitreal triamcinolone for uveitic cystoid macular edema: an optical coherence tomography study. Ophthalmology 2001; 108(4):765–772.
4. Ferrante P, Ramsey A, Bunce C, et al. Clinical trial to compare efficacy and side-effects of injection of posterior sub-Tenon triamcinolone versus orbital floor methylprednisolone in the management of posterior uveitis. Clin Experiment Ophthalmol 2004; 32(6):563–568.
5. Weijtens O, Feron EJ, Schoemaker RC, et al. High concentration of dexamethasone in aqueous and vitreous after subconjunctival injection. Am J Ophthalmol 1999; 128(2):192–197.
6. Weijtens O, Schoemaker RC, Cohen AF, et al. Dexamethasone concentration in vitreous and serum after oral administration. Am J Ophthalmol 1998; 125(5):673–679.

7. Weijtens O, van der Sluijs FA, Schoemaker RC, et al. Peribulbar corticosteroid injection: vitreal and serum concentrations after dexamethasone disodium phosphate injection. Am J Ophthalmol 1997; 123(3):358–363.

8. Imrie FR, Dick AD. Nonsteroidal drugs for the treatment of noninfectious posterior and intermediate uveitis. Curr Opin Ophthalmol 2007; 18(3):212–219.

9. Okada AA. Immunomodulatory therapy for ocular inflammatory disease: a basic manual and review of the literature. Ocul Immunol Inflamm 2005; 13(5):335–351.

10. Thorne JE, Jabs DA, Qazi FA, et al. Mycophenolate mofetil therapy for inflammatory eye disease. Ophthalmology 2005; 112(8):1472–1477.

11. Hogan AC, McAvoy CE, Dick AD, et al. Long-term efficacy and tolerance of tacrolimus for the treatment of uveitis. Ophthalmology 2007; 114(5):1000–1006.

12. Samson CM, Waheed N, Baltatzis S, et al. Methotrexate therapy for chronic noninfectious uveitis: analysis of a case series of 160 patients. Ophthalmology 2001; 108(6):1134–1139.

13. Baker KB, Spurrier NJ, Watkins AS, et al. Retention time for corticosteroid-sparing systemic immunosuppressive agents in patients with inflammatory eye disease. Br J Ophthalmol 2006; 90(12):1481–1485.

14. Foeldvari I, Nielsen S, Kummerle-Deschner J, et al. Tumor necrosis factor-alpha blocker in treatment of juvenile idiopathic arthritis-associated uveitis refractory to second-line agents: results of a multinational survey. J Rheumatol 2007; 34(5): 1146–11450.

15. Jabs DA, Nussenblatt RB, Rosenbaum JT. Standardization of uveitis nomenclature for reporting clinical data. Results of the First International Workshop. Am J Ophthalmol 2005; 140(3):509–516.

16. Nussenblatt RB, Palestine AG, Chan CC, et al. Standardization of vitreal inflammatory activity in intermediate and posterior uveitis. Ophthalmology 1985; 92(4):467–471.

17. Murphy CC, Hughes EH, Frost NA, et al. Quality of life and visual function in patients with intermediate uveitis. Br J Ophthalmol 2005; 89(9):1161–1165.

18. Becker MD, Smith JR, Max R, et al. Management of sight-threatening uveitis: new therapeutic options. Drugs 2005; 65(4):497–519.

5
Immunomodulatory Therapy

As has been highlighted in chapter 4, the treatment of posterior segment intraocular inflammation (PSII) requires an individualized approach based on the particular disease process, severity, systemic manifestations, age, sex, and medical history of each patient. Determining appropriate treatment requires experience and knowledge of the action and safety of the drugs we use, more so because it requires a process of drug trial and suitable and timely amendments to therapy. For example, specific agents may be started then discontinued due to inadequate efficacy, onset of adverse effects, or with the plan to only use the agent for a short period of time while waiting for a second agent to "kick in." Sometimes treatments are initiated as a "diagnostic trial" in patients without an established diagnosis. Ineffectiveness of a treatment may indicate either that a presumed diagnosis is incorrect or it may merely mean that there has been inadequate immunosuppression (e.g., not high enough dosage; requires a change to more potent immunosuppressive agent or requires triple therapy). Such management issues have been covered in previous chapters.

This chapter will describe systemic immunomodulatory agents used in the treatment of noninfectious intraocular inflammation. The implication is that active infectious disease has been ruled out as a cause of the intraocular inflammation, although in some cases we do use immunomodulatory agents in addition to antimicrobial drugs for certain infectious diseases (e.g., the use of corticosteroids to reduce retinal damage due to severe inflammation in acute retinal necrosis and *Toxoplasma* chorioretinitis). However, by and large, this chapter will address the use of immunomodulatory drugs to treat presumed autoimmune or autoinflammatory disease of the eye. A section on the use of periocular and intravitreal administration of corticosteroids is also added, as this may be useful for acute inflammatory recurrences. Finally, since uveitis often generates structural damage necessitating surgery (including cataract, glaucoma, and vitreoretinal procedures), a section is included on perioperative medical management to maximize the outcome for patients by preventing unwanted inflammatory relapses.

WHAT IS IMMUNOMODULATORY THERAPY?

Immunomodulatory therapy (IMT) encompasses treatment based on drugs that modulate the immune system. This includes an ever-increasing variety of agents, starting with those that nonspecifically inhibit inflammation and induce a degree of immunosuppression, such as corticosteroids, to drugs that are used for their widespread immunosuppressive effect, such as methotrexate, to agents that specifically inhibit T cells such as cyclosporin A. Furthermore, we are now seeing an explosion of development in preclinical tests and phase 1 clinical trials of a category of drugs called "biologic agents." (Currently there a four in clinical use in uveitis and 22 under study.) These are usually aimed at manipulating a specific cytokine's or chemokine's activity, either by augmenting the molecule as in the case of interferon-α (IFN-α) or inhibiting the molecule as in the case of tumor necrosis factor-α (TNF-α) (infliximab). Biologic agents can also be designed to manipulate other naturally occurring molecules, such as cellular adhesion molecules. These biologic agents have been quickly adopted into the overall IMT strategy and have started to alter our way of thinking in terms of treatment. A traditional approach to treatment of inflammatory diseases is to start out with less powerful drugs having few adverse effects and then escalate treatment to stronger agents if inflammation is not contained. This has several problems. By doing so we may be undertreating sight-threatening disease. However, also as highlighted by the move to recent approaches to treatment, in conditions with poorly predictable outcomes, treating with more potent immunosuppressive agents may prevent tissue damage altogether.

Box 1 summarizes both views, with the traditional thinking being called the "step-up" approach and the new thinking being referred to as the "top-down" approach.

Our rheumatology colleagues have been at the forefront of developing the top-down approach (1), and are currently comparing the two approaches in a randomized clinical trial in patients with recent onset Crohn's disease (2). The possibility exists that, not only will significant tissue damage be avoided, but patients receiving top-down treatment may also experience higher rates of remission, which of course is the ultimate goal. Many uveitis specialists are also believers in the

Box 1　Algorithm of Two Approaches to Immunomodulation

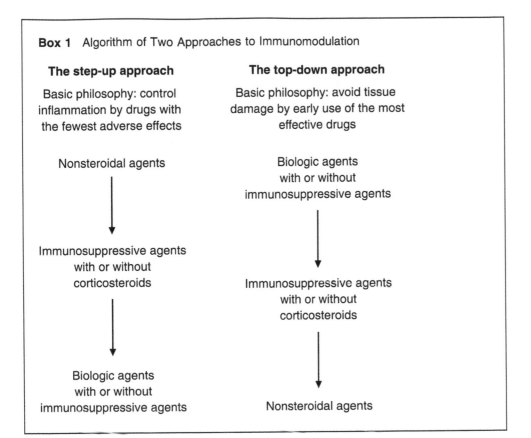

The step-up approach	The top-down approach
Basic philosophy: control inflammation by drugs with the fewest adverse effects	Basic philosophy: avoid tissue damage by early use of the most effective drugs
Nonsteroidal agents	Biologic agents with or without immunosuppressive agents
Immunosuppressive agents with or without corticosteroids	Immunosuppressive agents with or without corticosteroids
Biologic agents with or without immunosuppressive agents	Nonsteroidal agents

top-down strategy. After all, why wait for the patient to go blind if you already know that the visual prognosis of a certain disease (a good example would be Behçet's disease) is poor? However, it must be noted that the top-down approach has yet to undergo the scrutiny of a randomized controlled trial in uveitis. In addition, the use of biologic agents with potentially severe adverse effects requires a great deal of understanding on the part of the patient, as well as a degree of experience and expertise on the part of the physicians involved. Nevertheless, you could interpret that uveitis specialists already, in the presence of sight-threatening ocular inflammation (STOI), engage a top-down approach by instituting high-dose corticosteroid therapy alongside early introduction of IMT.

With the caveat that our IMT strategies are in the midst of evolving, this chapter will present the major IMT agents used for PSII in historical order, starting with corticosteroids, moving on to immunosuppressive agents and ending with biologic agents. The reader is also encouraged to refer frequently back to chapters 2 and 4 for generic treatment algorithms, a general discussion on pretreatment investigations, how to select an IMT agent, monitoring of response to treatment, and monitoring for adverse effects.

CORTICOSTEROIDS

Decades ago, the knee-jerk response to therapy in chronic noninfectious uveitis was to start with systemic corticosteroids *and* often continue this for a long period of time. Thankfully, today, greater experience and availability of a wider variety of effective treatment modalities help us to avoid such treatment and the myriad of adverse effects associated with it. Regardless, the relatively short-term use of systemic corticosteroids or the longer-term use of systemic corticosteroids at low doses in combination with immunosuppressive agents does remain a mainstay in the treatment of uveitic diseases with severe acute onset or chronic/recurrent inflammation. Although this is true for many PSII, particularly notable examples include Vogt-Koyanagi-Harada (VKH) disease, sympathetic ophthalmia, Behçet's disease, and birdshot chorioretinopathy.

The mechanism of action involves binding of drug to specific cytoplasmic steroid receptors that are present in virtually every cell of the body. The corticosteroid-receptor complex then enters the nucleus, binds to DNA at specific sites, and either promotes or inhibits the transcription of numerous genes. The end result is not only broad suppression of inflammation and the immune response but also broad effects on the hypothalamic-pituitary-adrenal axis; metabolism of carbohydrates, proteins, and lipids; regulation of electrolytes; bone metabolism; and functioning of the central nervous and cardiovascular systems.

Because of such far-reaching influences on the body, the systemic use of corticosteroids is associated with a myriad of adverse effects, particularly if used chronically. The major adverse effects are summarized in Table 1 and relative contraindications for this treatment modality are listed in Table 2.

In order to avoid inevitable long-term adverse effects, systemic corticosteroids should be tapered as soon as possible, but without causing a recurrence in disease activity. If one is confident that the corticosteroids can be tapered off entirely within six months to a year for the disease one is treating, as may be the case for acute VKH disease, *and* there are no complicating medical factors such as diabetes mellitus or osteoporosis, then there is usually no need to use a second agent. However, if long-term therapy is anticipated for chronic disease, then a second steroid-sparing IMT agent should be considered either at the beginning of the treatment with corticosteroids or when the corticosteroid dose is tapered to 20 to 30 mg/day prednisolone or equivalent (a methodology also referred to as "combination therapy" (see Fig. 10 of chap. 2). As was suggested by a multinational panel of uveitis experts, the overall aim should be to avoid using much more than 10 mg of prednisolone or equivalent for chronic therapy (3). The reader should also refer to the discussion in chapter 4 regarding "instituting systemic steroid therapy" for noninfectious STOI.

A typical dose for oral corticosteroids for the initial treatment of an active disease process would be 1.0 to 1.5 mg/kg/day of prednisolone or equivalent. Initial therapy involving IV corticosteroids, often administered as a pulse dose (e.g., methylprednisolone 1000 mg/day for 3 days) followed by oral cortico-steroids, is commonly used in regions of the world for the treatment of VKH disease (4) and several other conditions (see chap. 4).

IMMUNOSUPPRESSIVE AGENTS

Immunosuppressive agents encompass a wide variety of drugs that suppress immune cells via a few basic mechanisms: interfering with a metabolite essential to nucleotide synthesis (the antimetabolites), causing cellular death by damaging DNA (the alkylating agents), or inhibiting T-cell activation (the T-cell inhibitors). Immunosuppressive agents have formed the backbone of our treatment of posterior or panuveitis, particularly in cases of STOI. Furthermore, their role in allowing us to reduce systemic corticosteroid use is equally important, particularly in patients who are elderly or have comorbidities such as diabetes mellitus. In general, the antimetabolites or T-cell inhibitors are favored over the alkylating agents because of the association of the latter with secondary malignancies. The drugs most commonly used in ocular inflammation are noted in Box 2 and are described below.

The reader should also refer to chapter 4 for details on pretreatment investigations, mandatory in order to rule out conditions that may increase the risk

Table 1 Major Adverse Effects of Systemically Administered Corticosteroids

Infectious	Skin	Gastrointestinal	Endocrine	Musculoskeletal	Central nervous system	Ophthalmic
Opportunistic infection	Thinning or fragility	Nonspecific upset	Glucose intolerance	Myopathy	Mood alteration	Glaucoma
Impaired wound healing	Acne	Gastritis or peptic ulcer if NSAIDs also used	Diabetes mellitus	Osteoporosis	Insomnia	Cataract
	Hirsutism	Pancreatitis	Hypolipoproteinemia	Compression fracture	Depression	
	Ecchymoses		Fat redistribution	Aseptic necrosis of the femoral head	Psychosis	
			Hypothalamic-pituitary-adrenal axis suppression	Growth suppression in children	Pseudotumor cerebri	
			Acute adrenal insufficiency			

Abbreviation: NSAIDs, nonsteroidal anti-inflammatory drugs.

Table 2 Relative Contraindications of Systemically
Administered Corticosteroids

"When to think about whether it is safe to use steroids"

Active systemic infection
History of tuberculosis
HIV infection
Pregnancy
Growing children
Diabetes mellitus
Uncontrolled hypertension
Embolic disease
Osteoporosis
History of compression fracture
Clinical depression
Psychiatric disease

**Box 2   Commonly used immunosuppressive agents in ocular inflammatory
disease**

Antimetabolites:	Azathioprine
	Methotrexate
	Mycophenolate mofetil
Alkylating agents:	Cyclophosphamide
T-cell inhibitors:	Cyclosporin A
	Tacrolimus

---

of developing adverse effects. Furthermore, although some experienced uveitis
specialists feel comfortable with prescribing IMT and monitoring for adverse
effects, consultation with appropriate internal medicine specialists should be
considered, particularly for patients with comorbidities and for children.

Azathioprine

Azathioprine is one of the more commonly used immunosuppressive agents
because of its mild adverse effect profile. A few case series have shown that
azathioprine, used in conjunction with low-dose corticosteroids, was successful in
controlling posterior intraocular inflammation involving a variety of noninfectious

diseases such as Behçet's disease, serpiginous choroidopathy, multifocal choroiditis and panuveitis, and noninfectious neuroretinitis (5). Furthermore, a two-year randomized, placebo-controlled, double-blind trial in Turkish men with Behçet's disease showed that azathioprine at 2.5 mg/kg/day reduced ocular involvement (6).

- *Mechanism of action*: Azathioprine is a purine analog converted by the liver to 6-mercaptopurine and then to thiopurine nucleotides, which represent the active compounds. These thiopurine nucleotides interfere with de novo synthesis of purine nucleotides and are also directly incorporated into DNA and RNA, ultimately causing a decrease in circulating lymphocytes, suppression of lymphocyte proliferation, and inhibition of antibody production.
- *Contraindications*: Individuals with low or absent thiopurine methyltransferase (TPMT), one of the enzymes involved in the liver metabolism of this drug. Unfortunately, testing for TPMT activity is not widely available. Other contraindications are pregnancy and women attempting to get pregnant.
- *Dosage*: 1 to 3 mg/kg/day orally.
- *Adverse effects*: Gastrointestinal symptoms occur in 15% to 30% of patients involving nausea, vomiting, or diarrhea (7). Myelosuppression usually occurs at higher doses than recommended in ocular inflammation; however, low-dose azathioprine therapy (1–2 mg/kg/day) resulted in leukopenia in 4.5% and thrombocytopenia in 2% of rheumatoid arthritis patients in one study (7). Patients who develop myelosuppression may have low or absent TPMT activity. Other adverse effects include mild hepatic dysfunction, increased risk of infections, possible increased risk of malignancy, and drug hypersensitivity. Since data on teratogenicity is limited, azathioprine should be avoided in pregnancy.
- *Monitoring*: Complete blood counts (CBC) and liver function tests every four to six weeks.

Methotrexate

Methotrexate is also a favored IMT agent due to its relatively benign adverse effect profile (at low doses), as well as its long track record in other autoinflammatory diseases such as rheumatoid arthritis and juvenile idiopathic arthritis (JIA). However, definite teratogenicity limits its use in women of childbearing age. Several case series have shown methotrexate to be effective in patients either unresponsive to or intolerant of corticosteroid therapy in a wide variety of posterior intraocular inflammatory diseases, including sarcoidosis, Behçet's disease, VKH disease, and multifocal choroiditis and panuveitis (5). However, randomized controlled trials evaluating methotrexate therapy have not been performed specifically in ocular inflammation. Therefore, whether methotrexate is beneficial is less certain compared to other immunosuppressives. Many of the reported studies addressed control of systemic inflammation where there was a clear beneficial effect. However, in the context of JIA-associated uveitis, it is not clear that many of the patients under study would have developed significant ocular disease in the first place (8).

- *Mechanism of action*: Methotrexate is a folic acid analog that inactivates dihydrofolate reductase (DHFR), resulting in the inhibition of folic acid metabolism that ultimately inhibits the synthesis of purines and thymidylate. Methotrexate also inhibits folate-dependent enzymes. Folinic acid (leucovorin) is a folate coenzyme that restores thymidylate and purine even in the presence of methotrexate and is also used to "rescue" normal cells from toxicity with high doses of methotrexate, as used in cancer treatment. In ocular inflammatory disease, generally only low doses are used. Methotrexate and all its metabolites are excreted in the urine.
- *Contraindications*: Folic acid deficiency, renal disease, liver disease, pregnancy, women attempting to get pregnant.
- *Dosage*: Therapy should start at doses of 5 to 7.5 mg/wk and gradually increased to 15 to 20 mg/wk depending on the clinical response. However, efficacy of starting at 25 mg/wk for inflammatory bowel disease again supports its use at higher doses initially to control inflammation. This has not been taken on board by ophthalmologists. The drug may be administered orally or by subcutaneous, intramuscular, or intravenous injections. Oral administration may be associated with variable bioavailability. Folic acid at 1 mg/day should be given to reduce gastrointestinal toxicity and myelosuppression. Folinic acid at 5 mg/wk may also be administered 8 to 12 hours before or after the methotrexate dose. Subcutaneous routes may allow lower doses to maintain efficacy and reduce adverse effects, particularly useful in the management of JIA.
- *Adverse effects:* The major concern is myelosuppression, and occurs in approximately 5% of rheumatoid arthritis patients undergoing low-dose therapy (9). Gastrointestinal disturbances such as nausea, vomiting, and diarrhea are common at the initiation of treatment. Hepatotoxicity may occur in 15% of patients, and patients with hepatitis B or C infection, known liver disease, or a history of alcoholism should undergo a baseline liver biopsy before considering methotrexate treatment (5). Other adverse effects include skin disturbances such as urticaria and cutaneous vasculitis, central nervous system toxicity, pulmonary toxicity, osteoporosis, and opportunistic infection. Lymphoproliferative disorders have been reported, and because methotrexate is a known teratogen, it must not

be used in pregnant women. Overall, this immunosuppressive is arguably the better tolerated, but potentially at the expense of efficacy.

- *Monitoring*: CBC, serum creatinine and liver function tests every one to two months.

Mycophenolate Mofetil (Cellcept)

There is somewhat less experience with the use of mycophenolate mofetil compared to the other antimetabolites. However, the drug is generally well tolerated, and several case series have reported mycophenolate mofetil to be effective in patients who have failed therapy using cyclosporin A and/or azathioprine in combination with low-dose corticosteroids (5). A retrospective study of 84 patients with uveitis, scleritis, or other ocular inflammatory disease found that mycophenolate was effective as a steroid-sparing agent, with manageable adverse effects, the most common being gastrointestinal upset (10).

- *Mechanism of action*: Mycophenolate mofetil inhibits inosine monophosphate dehydrogenase, which is necessary for the de novo synthesis of purines. Lymphocytes are particularly dependent on de novo purine synthesis and therefore mycophenolate mofetil has a relative selectivity for suppressing T- and B-cell proliferation.
- *Contraindications*: Pregnancy, women attempting to get pregnant.
- *Dosage*: 0.5 to 1.5 grams twice a day orally.
- *Adverse effects*: The most common adverse effects are gastrointestinal disturbances such as diarrhea, nausea, and abdominal pain. Malignancies and opportunistic infections have been reported. Data on teratogenicity is limited, and therefore mycophenolate mofetil should be avoided in pregnancy.
- *Monitoring:* When initiating treatment, a CBC should be checked every week for one month, every two weeks for two months, then monthly thereafter. Liver function tests should be added every three months.

Cyclophosphamide

Cyclophosphamide was one of the early IMT agents to be used in rheumatology and ocular inflammatory disease. However, the use of alkylating agents such as cyclophosphamide (and previously chlorambucil) are associated with an increased risk of secondary malignancies. Today, the alkylating agents are usually selected only after failure using therapy with antimetabolites. In the case of cyclophosphamide, the specific risk of bladder cancer must be discussed with patients and periodic bladder cancer screening must be performed for life. In addition, the adverse effect of cyclophosphamide on subsequent fertility in both men and women must be made clear to the patient. The rate of sustained amenorrhea after cyclophosphamide therapy for autoinflammatory disease ranges from 11% to 59% and ovarian failure is common, particularly in women of older ages and with larger cumulative doses (11). There is less data on men; however, one study in patients with Behçet's disease being treated with cyclophosphamide found that azoospermia or severe oligospermia developed in 13 of 17 men (12). Therefore, prior to initiation of cyclophosphamide treatment, specific counseling and the opportunity for ova or sperm banking should be provided. Cyclophosphamide is also associated with profound immunosuppression, and secondary infections such as CMV and *Pneumocystis* pneumonia (see below) are not infrequent.

In terms of efficacy, IV cyclosphosphamide therapy has been used for various uveitidies with mixed results (5,13). One study in Behçet's disease patients found pulse IV cyclosphosphamide to be inferior to cyclosporin A (14). Retrospective analysis of a large number of patients with Behçet's disease also found combination therapy using cyclophosphamide and colchicine to be inferior to therapy involving cyclosporin A (15). Thus, given the significant risks associated with use of this drug, the lack of data showing efficacy, and the growing use of biologic agents, cyclophophamide is likely to play an extremely limited role in the future of IMT.

- *Mechanism of action*: Cyclophosphamide is an analog of nitrogen mustard, metabolized by the liver into several active compounds that alkylate purine bases, resulting in inhibition of DNA and RNA synthesis and function.
- *Contraindications*: Bladder dysfunction, pregnancy, women attempting to get pregnant.
- *Dosage*: Oral therapy is usually initiated at a dose of 1 to 3 mg/kg/day. Pulse IV therapy is at an initial dose of 500 mg/M^2 of body surface area. This is then repeated every four weeks, depending on the clinical response and white blood cell count. The dose should be reduced for white blood cell counts of less than 2000/mm^3 (13). Studies in lupus nephritis show little difference in adverse events between oral and IV treatments.
- *Adverse effects*: Myelosuppression is the most common adverse effect, although the degree of leukopenia is used in many cases as a marker for immunosuppressive effect. Opportunistic infections such as *Pneumocystis* pneumonia may occur with chronic therapy, even at low doses. Bladder toxicity may result in hemorrhagic cystitis or bladder cancer and, therefore, patients should maintain adequate hydration (16). Adverse

effects include other secondary malignancies, opportunistic infections, gastrointestinal upset, alopecia, and pneumonitis. Cyclophosphamide is a teratogen and must not be used in pregnant women.

- *Monitoring:* When initiating therapy, CBC, platelet count, and urinalysis should be checked once a week, then monthly when stable.

Cyclosporin A

Cyclosporin A is probably the most widely used IMT agent for ocular inflammatory disease due to its relatively mild toxicity profile and its efficacy in diseases with STOI, particularly Behçet's disease. Both cyclosporin A and tacrolimus specifically inhibit T cells and therefore have little myelosuppression; however, nephrotoxicity often limits their use in patients. Cyclosporin A has been shown to be superior to combination corticosteroid and chlorambucil therapy (17) and also superior to colchicine (18) in two separate randomized controlled trials of patients with Behçet's disease. However, one must be aware that the doses used in these clinical trials were higher than what is generally used today. Other randomized studies and numerous case series have also reported efficacy with cyclosporin A in patients with a variety of noninfectious uveitis, usually in combination with low-dose corticosteroids (5).

- *Mechanism of action*: Cyclosporine A is a calcineurin inhibitor and complexes with an intracellular binding protein called cyclophilin, which in turn binds to calcineurin and inhibits translocation of cytosolic nuclear factor of activated T cells. The result is interference in transcription of genes for T cell activation. Cyclosporin A is metabolized in the liver and excreted in bile. It has a high volume of distribution accumulating in body fat.
- *Contraindications:* Renal disease, pregnancy, women attempting to get pregnant.
- *Dosage*: 3 to 5 mg/kg/day.
- *Adverse effects*: Renal toxicity is dose dependent, and generally reversible. However, irreversible toxicity may occur if serum creatinine levels rise to greater than 50% over baseline, and there is some evidence to suggest that renal toxicity may be avoided if doses are kept below 4 mg/kg/day (19). Other adverse effects include hypertension, gastrointestinal upset, hypertrichosis, gingival hyperplasia, tremor, paresthesia, breast tenderness, hyperkalemia, hypomagnesemia, hypercholesterolemia, and elevated uric acid. At the doses used in rheumatologic and ocular inflammatory diseases, secondary malignancies have not occurred. Data on teratogenicity is limited, and therefore cyclosporin A should be

avoided in pregnancy. Finally, although widely used for ocular involvement in Behçet's disease, there is some data to suggest that the development of central nervous system abnormalities may be associated with cyclosporin A therapy (20), although it is unclear whether this is a manifestation of drug toxicity or of the disease itself.

- *Monitoring*: Blood pressure and the serum creatinine should be checked every two weeks when initiating therapy, then monthly when stable. Electrolytes, magnesium, and uric acid should also be monitored monthly, and the cholesterol profile every three months. Cyclosporin A drug levels may be measured to judge bioavailability, although this may not correlate with clinical efficacy.

Tacrolimus

Compared with cyclosporin A, there is less experience reported using tacrolimus in ocular inflammatory disease. However, a randomized study found that, while both drugs were equally effective in uveitis, tacrolimus was associated with fewer adverse effects, particularly the cardiovascular disease risk factors of hypertension and hypercholesterolemia (21). This was also found to be true in renal transplant patients undergoing immunosuppressive therapy (22). Thus, patients already on cyclosporin A, in whom long-term therapy is anticipated, may benefit from conversion to tacrolimus. Furthermore, a long-term follow-up study in 62 consecutive patients receiving tacrolimus for uveitis found that 85% achieved tapering of oral prednisolone to a dose of less than or equal to 10 mg/day after one year two months of treatment (23). This study also confirmed the relatively low rate of adverse effects.

- *Mechanism of action*: Tacrolimus (FK-506) is also a calcineurin inhibitor but is structurally different from cyclosporin A and binds to a different intracellular binding protein called FK-binding protein. This complex then associates with calcineurin and induces the same action as cyclosporin A, resulting in interference of T-cell activation.
- *Contraindications*: Renal disease, pregnancy, women attempting to get pregnant.
- *Dosage*: 0.05 to 0.15 mg/kg/day. Dose can be titrated to trough (12 hour post-dose) serum levels (aim between 5 and 10 ng/mL).
- *Adverse effects*: Same as for cyclosporin A; however, with lower rates of hypertension and hypercholesterolemia (21,22). Data on teratogenicity is limited, and therefore tacrolimus should be avoided in pregnancy. Also consider alternative immunosuppression in patients with impaired glucose tolerance or diabetes mellitus.
- *Monitoring:* Same as for cyclosporin A.

BIOLOGIC AGENTS

The biologic agents are a completely new category of IMT, with the goal of manipulating the activity of a variety of naturally occurring substances, in particular cytokines (24). Biologic agents have met with great success in a variety of autoinflammatory diseases, such as rheumatoid arthritis, psoriatic arthritis, inflammatory bowel disease, and multiple sclerosis. Their use in ocular inflammatory disease remains limited to "refractory" disease or in the specific case of Behçet's disease, the latter due to its high risk of STOI.

Interferon-α

IFN-α, although technically speaking a biologic agent, is not a new drug, having been available on the market as a therapeutic agent since the early 1980s. In fact, IFN-α was the first cytokine to be successfully manufactured using recombinant technology and is used today in a variety of diseases, most prominently chronic hepatitis B and C infection for its antiviral effect, and also in a variety of cancers such as chronic myelogenous leukemia and AIDS-related Kaposi's sarcoma. The use of IFN-α in uveitis started in the 1990s when Behçet's patients were treated, under the hypothesis that some sort of viral process was contributing to the pathogenesis of oral aphthous ulcers and genital lesions. These patients were found to have improvement not only in their mucocutaneous lesions but also in their uveitis (25,26). A prospective, open-label trial specifically conducted in Behçet's disease patients with uveitis showed that the drug was effective in suppressing inflammatory attacks as well as improving visual acuity (27), and these results have been confirmed in several retrospective studies in Behçet's disease and other types of noninfectious posterior and panuveitis as well (28–30). However, perhaps due to such "immunomodulatory" effects, patients treated with IFN-α may also have adverse effects in the form of a variety of autoinflammatory phenomena such as development of antinuclear antibodies and antithyroid antibodies, as well as frank onset of autoinflammatory disorders such as systemic lupus erythematosus and Hashimoto thyroiditis.

- *Mechanism of action*: IFN-α has antiviral, antitumor, antiangiogenic, and immunomodulatory properties; however, its specific mechanism of action in Behçet's disease is unclear at this time. IFN-α and the structurally related IFN-β are both type I IFNs that share the same cell surface receptor associated with tyrosine kinase 2. Binding to this receptor induces rapid tyrosine phosphorylation of the receptor and subsequent induction of transcription of a set of genes called IFN-stimulated genes, including those for protein kinase R (which regulates cellular and viral protein synthesis), Mx proteins (that have antiviral actions), and proteins with antioncogene expression. IFN-α has been shown in patients receiving treatment for Behçet's disease to promote induction of IL-10 producing T cells that may be serving as regulatory T cells (31).

- *Contraindications*: Clinical depression or other psychiatric disease, HIV infection, other active infection, liver disease, renal disease, cardiovascular disease, thyroid dysfunction, autoinflammatory disease, coagulopathy, pregnancy, women attempting to get pregnant.

- *Dosage*: 3 to 6 million IU by subcutaneous injection, daily to three times per week. Dose should be adjusted and tapered to reach minimum effective dose. Dose can also be tapered to reduce adverse effects, particularly fatigue. In addition, the beneficial effects of IFN-α may be inhibited by use of other immunosuppression. Therefore, most patients require a washout period before commencing IFN-α therapy (30). There are two randomized clinical trials yet to be reported. There is no data to confirm which recombinant IFN-α (recombinant IFN-α2A or liposomal recombinant IFN-α2B) is more beneficial in ocular disease.

- *Adverse effects*: Flu-like symptoms, generalized fatigue and asthenia, arrhythmia, cardiomyopathy, clinical depression including suicidal behavior, paresthesias, other central nervous system dysfunction, gastrointestinal disturbances, hepatotoxicity, pneumonitis, alopecia, retinal hemorrhages and cotton wool spots, and onset or exacerbation of a variety of autoinflammatory disorders including thyroiditis, thrombocytopenia, Raynaud's phenomenon, rheumatoid arthritis, and systemic lupus erythematosus. Data on the use of IFN-α in pregnancy is limited and therefore should be avoided.

- *Monitoring*: Initially weekly CBC and platelet counts, then monthly once stable alongside biochemistry and liver function tests.

Infliximab

Infliximab is a chimeric monoclonal antibody against TNF-α and is one of several biologic agents developed to block TNF-α action. TNF-α is a proinflammatory cytokine known to be elevated in a variety of autoinflammatory diseases, including rheumatoid arthritis, Crohn's disease, and ankylosing spondylitis, and efficacy of infliximab has been shown for these diseases (32–34). In ophthalmology, infliximab has been reported to effectively control inflammation associated with a variety of posterior uveitidies, including sarcoidosis, pars planitis, and Behçet's disease, as well as in anterior uveitis and scleritis (35–37). Futhermore, many patients with Behçet's disease have experienced a complete halt in inflammatory attacks (38–40). Yet our experience in ocular inflammatory diseases remains preliminary. It is also unclear whether infliximab is capable of inducing remission as defined by the Standardization of Uveitis Nomenclature (SUN) guidelines as "greater than 3 months of inactivity off all therapy" (41). One of the most important indications for infliximab use is turning out to be Behçet's disease. However, this disease tends to occur at higher incidences in parts of the world that also have higher incidences of tuberculosis, recrudescence of which is one of the major adverse effects observed with infliximab therapy (42). Potentially fatal adverse effects also include other opportunistic infections, central nervous system dysfunction, and thromboembolic events (43). It is unclear whether concomitant immunosuppressive agents, such as methotrexate or azathioprine as used in rheumatoid arthritis or Crohn's disease patients on infliximab therapy, are beneficial in order to avoid development of anti-infliximab antibodies and perhaps prolong the therapeutic response (44). Therefore, while infliximab therapy is an extremely promising IMT agent, more experience is necessary to delineate its appropriate use in the treatment of patients with ocular inflammatory disease.

- *Mechanism of action*: Infliximab not only binds to soluble TNF-α, preventing the interaction of TNF-α with its cell surface receptor, but also binds to membrane-bound TNF-α, resulting in cytotoxicity to TNF-α-expressing cells. This cytotoxic effect is not observed with the other TNF-α blockers.
- *Contraindications*: Active or recent serious infection, HIV infection, chronic infection such as with hepatitis B or hepatitis C virus, untreated active or latent tuberculosis (screening is imperative prior to commencing therapy), thromboembolic disease, congestive heart failure, multiple sclerosis or other demyelinating disorder, recent malignancy, history of lymphoma, history of organ transplantation, pregnancy, women attempting to get pregnant, known allergy to murine or chimeric proteins.
- *Dosage*: 5 mg/kg intravenously. The treatment protocol for Behçet's disease and diseases such as rheumatoid arthritis and Crohn's disease involves administering infusions at weeks 0, 2, and 6, followed by an infusion every eight weeks.
- *Adverse effects*: Infusion reaction (itching, flushing, nausea, dyspnea, hypotension, or hypertension), injection site reactions (erythema, itching, swelling), opportunistic infections especially upper respiratory tract infections, new or reactivation of tuberculosis, bacterial infections, development of anticardiolipin antibodies and/or other autoantibodies, myocardial infarction, pulmonary embolism, other embolic disorders,

non-Hodgkin's lymphoma, other malignancies, demyelinating disease, drug-induced lupus. Data on the use of infliximab in pregnancy is limited and thus should be avoided.

- *Monitoring*: CBC, electrolytes, creatinine, liver function tests, creatine kinase, and C-reactive protein just prior to each infusion.

Other Biologic Agents

As has already been observed in systemic autoinflammatory disease, not all patients will respond to the same drug, and one drug is rarely a "cure" for any disease. For example, there is growing evidence indicating that rheumatoid arthritis patients who fail infliximab therapy may respond to other TNF-α inhibitors (45). In the field of ocular inflammation, the TNF receptor 2 (TNFR2) immunofusion protein, etanercept, which can bind to both TNF-α and TNF-β and lymphotoxin, has limited evidence for efficacy despite a positive study in treatment-resistant chronic anterior uveitis in children (46). These results are not surprising as experimental animal models show that most TNF-driven ocular inflammation is TNFR1 dependent, which etanercept does not target. In addition, etanercept has been linked to de novo ocular inflammation, including uveitis and scleritis. On the other hand, adalimumab, the recombinant humanized monoclonal antibody against TNF-α, has similar action to infliximab, and not surprisingly is efficacious in Behçet's disease with ocular manifestations (47) and chronic anterior uveitis in children (48).

The explosion in biotechnology and engineering has furnished us with numerous other biologic factors, other than TNF-α, which have and may be targeted in the future. For example, a small study using the anti-CD52 monoclonal antibody campath-1H also reported efficacy in Behçet's disease by means of depleting CD4$^+$ T cells, although two patients developed hypothyroidism as an adverse effect (49). The utility of campath-1H for the uveitis of Behçet's disease was not specifically addressed in this study. campath-1H showed remarkable efficacy in a small cohort of noninfectious ocular inflammatory diseases of various etiology (50). The use of daclizumab, a humanized monoclonal antibody against the IL-2 receptor, has been found in a short-term, open-label, multicenter clinical trial of patients with noninfectious uveitis to be safe and possibly associated with reduction in need for concomitant immuno-suppressive therapy (51). Anakinra, a humanized monoclonal antibody against the IL-1 receptor, was successfully used in one patient with posterior uveitis associated with chronic infantile neurologic cutaneous articular (CINCA) syndrome (52). Finally, abatacept (fusion protein that binds the costimulatory factor B7, thereby inhibiting T-cell activation), rituximab (chimeric monoclonal antibody against CD20, widely expressed on B cells), and tocilizumab (humanized monoclonal antibody against IL-6) have all been found to have some efficacy in rheumatoid arthritis (45), and therefore may be under future consideration for patients with ocular inflammatory disease who fail other biologic agents. Indeed sporadic reports are trickling in from use in ophthalmology, and larger cohorts and trials are eagerly awaited. Clearly, the age of biologic therapy has only just begun, and we will continue to see a widening of our choice of treatment modalities in the years to come. Currently, most use of biologic agents is in patients who have "failed" conventional immunosuppression for a variety of reasons. In addition, a very wide range of ocular inflammatory diseases have been shown sporadically to have good effect from biologic therapy. Both these factors mitigate against the ease of conducting careful randomized clinical trials, but with the SUN guidelines in place it should be possible to initiate good multicenter trials and surveillance data, which may reveal that these agents have better effect if commenced earlier rather than later in treatment regimes—the top-down approach.

LOCALLY ADMINISTERED CORTICOSTEROIDS

In recent years, there has been a trend toward using periocular or intravitreal injections of corticosteroids in lieu of short-term systemic corticosteroids. However, this often trades potential systemic adverse effects for higher rates of the ocular adverse effects of cataract and glaucoma, particularly with intravitreal administration, and arguably less definitive and predictable long-term control of inflammation and outcome. A fluocinolone acetonide intravitreal implant was developed to reduce the need for long-term systemic therapy using corticosteroids and/or immunosuppressive agents; however, again this appears to be a trade-off between systemic and ocular adverse effects. We highlight some of the caveats to local corticosteroid therapy in chapter 4.

Periocular and Intravitreal Injections

The most common corticosteroid used for periocular injections is triamcinolone acetonide. Hydrocortisone, methylprednisolone, dexamethasone, and betamethasone are alternative agents. For PSII, transseptal injections, posterior sub-Tenon's injections, and retrobulbar injections are all effective. The standard dose for a

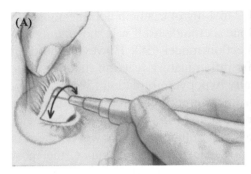 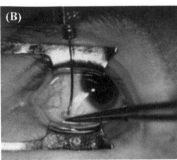

Figure 1 Two techniques for the administration of a posterior sub-Tenon's injection of triamcinolone acetonide are shown. **(A)** After topical anesthesia, a 25–gauge, 5/8-in sharp needle is inserted through conjunctiva into Tenon's capsule in the superotemporal quadrant of the globe with the patient looking down. The needle must be advanced to the hub to be able to inject in a posterior position. To ensure that globe penetration does not occur, this should be done while moving the tip of the needle slightly from side-to-side while checking for concomitant movement of the globe. If the globe moves together with the needle, then one infers that the point of the needle has engaged sclera and the needle should be withdrawn with an attempt to inject at a slightly different site. **(B)** Topical anesthesia is administered followed by standard prepping and draping. A small buttonhole incision is made through conjunctiva and Tenon's capsule approximately 10 mm posterior to the limbus in the inferotemporal quadrant, exposing bare sclera. A 23-gauge, curved blunt cannula, about 2.1 cm in length, is then inserted through the opening and advanced along the scleral surface to behind the globe, allowing injection of drug into a retrobulbar position. Suturing is not performed; however, topical antibiotics are used for one week after the injection, using this technique. *Source*: Figs. 1A, courtesy of Bausch and Lomb Inc.; 1B, courtesy of Kanehara Publishing Company.

transseptal injection (also referred to as orbital floor injection) of triamcinolone acetonide would be 40 mg in 1.0 cc, usually delivered through the temporal aspect of the lower lid. Posterior sub-Tenon's injections may require smaller doses of triamcinolone (e.g., 20 mg in 0.5 cc) and have higher efficacy (53). Two common techniques for delivering posterior sub-Tenon's injections are shown in Figure 1. For all periocular injections, particular care should be taken for eyes with high myopia and a long axial length, eyes status post–scleral buckling surgery, and eyes with scleral thinning due to scleritis or other causes.

Intravitreal injection of triamcinolone acetonide was advanced primarily by retinal specialists as a treatment for disease states such as macular edema due to retinal vein occlusion, diabetic macular edema, and exudative age-related macular degeneration (AMD) (54). This treatment has also come to be used by some uveitis specialists to treat refractory cystoid macular edema (CME) (55–57). As one might expect, efficacy appears to be higher with intravitreal injections over periocular injections. The standard dose is 2 to 4 mg of triamcinolone acetonide in a 0.05- to 0.1-cc injection. The triamcinolone acetonide itself was shown long ago to be nontoxic in a rabbit intravitreal injection model (58). However, the drug vehicle appears to potentiate a nonspecific inflammatory reaction in some eyes, with anterior chamber cells and occasionally hypopyon formation (59). This may depend on the specific drug formulation in different countries. Since the drug comes as a suspension, the vehicle can be separated from the drug particles, with the drug particles resuspended in balanced salt solution (60); however, there is no specific data to show how effective this maneuver is. Of course, the most devastating complication that can occur is infectious endophthalmitis, estimated to occur at a rate of 0.87% and includes infection with organisms that are difficult to detect and treat, such as *Mycobacterium chelonae* (61). It should be noted that the manufacturers of triamcinolone acetonide do not recommend this drug for intravitreal use, precisely because of the intraocular complications.

The adverse effects of all locally injected corticosteroids are listed in Table 3. The most common are cataract and glaucoma, both being dose-dependent adverse effects, occurring more frequently in eyes undergoing repeated injections. Corticosteroid-induced cataract and glaucoma develop at a particularly high rate with intravitreal injections, most likely due to the high dose of drug in proximity to the pertinent intraocular structures. One study involving 75 AMD eyes receiving a single intravitreal injection of 4 mg of triamcinolone acetonide found that 28% of eyes experienced an intraocular pressure (IOP) rise necessitating glaucoma medication and 29% of eyes followed for at least one year underwent

Table 3 Adverse Effects and Complications of Periocular or Intravitreal Injection of Corticosteroids

Periocular	Intravitreal	Both periocular and intravitreal
Inadvertent globe perforation	Inadvertent suprachoroidal space injection	Steroid-induced cataract
Optic nerve injury	Hypotony	Transient increased intraocular pressure
Lid ecchymosis	Vitreous hemorrhage	Glaucoma
Lid ptosis	Noninfective intraocular inflammation	Subconjunctival hemorrhage
Proptosis	Infective endophthalmitis	Injection site infection
Orbital fat atrophy	Traumatic cataract	Impaired glucose tolerance
Central retinal artery occlusion	Retinal tear	
	Retinal detachment	

Table 4 Relative Contraindications for Locally Administered Corticosteroids (Periocular Injection, Intravitreal Injection, Fluocinolone Acetonide Implant)

Active ocular infection
History of herpes keratitis or uveitis
History of cytomegalovirus retinitis or acute retinal necrosis
Glaucoma
Steroid responder
Advanced cataract

cataract surgery (62). It must also be noted that periocular and intravitreal corticosteroid injections do have some systemic absorption, and therefore may lead to poorer serum glucose control in patients with diabetes mellitus (see comments in chap. 4). Local injections of triamcinolone generally last for two to three months and therefore a repeat injection should not be considered before that time because of the increased risk of a rise in IOP. Relative contraindications for all locally administered corticosteroids are listed in Table 4.

Fluocinolone Acetonide Intravitreal Implant

The fluocinolone acetonide intravitreal implant was developed out of the great need to prolong anti-inflammatory efficacy over what was being achieved with periocular and/or intravitreal corticosteroid injections, while still avoiding major systemic adverse effects. The currently available device Retisert®, approved in the United States, is a scleral fixation drug delivery system containing 0.59-mg fluocinolone acetonide, designed to release therapeutic levels of drug over approximately 30 months (Fig. 2).

A multicenter randomized clinical trial in 278 patients with noninfectious posterior uveitis showed that, at 34 weeks of follow-up, the implant significantly reduced the number of uveitic recurrences, improved visual acuity, and decreased the need for adjunctive therapy such as systemic immunosuppression and periocular injections (63). However, this was associated with 51.1% of implanted eyes requiring IOP-lowering drops and 5.8% undergoing glaucoma filtering surgery. Furthermore, 9.9% of phakic implanted eyes had undergone cataract surgery by the end of the 34 week follow-up. An analysis of the pooled data from three multicenter clinical trials involving 584 implanted eyes showed that, over a three-year follow-up, 74.8% were administered IOP-lowering drops and 36.6% underwent glaucoma surgery (64).

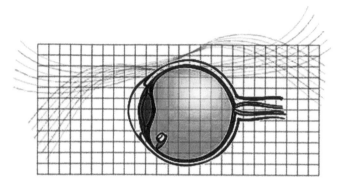

Figure 2 Retisert implant. The fluocinolone acetonide implant is scleral fixed as shown. Its slow release of corticosteroid into the vitreous is licensed for use for the treatment of noninfectious uveitis. *Source*: Courtesy of Bausch and Lomb Inc.

Glaucoma is clearly of prime concern in the use of this treatment modality. Other adverse effects that were somewhat unanticipated include the onset of cytomegalovirus retinitis in one patient with Behçet's disease (65), and vitreous band formation between the implant and the posterior pole, sometimes with macular traction requiring vitrectomy (66). The adverse effects of the fluocinolone acetonide implant are summarized in Table 5, and relative contraindications for all locally administered corticosteroids are listed in Table 4. In order to further delineate the role of the Retisert® implant in our clinics, the Multicenter Uveitis Steroid Treatment (MUST) trial is currently being performed to compare the efficacy of standard systemic therapy, including immunosuppression versus fluocinolone acetonide implant therapy, for the

Table 5 Adverse Effects and Complications of the Fluocinolone Acetonide Intravitreal Implant

Surgery-related problems	Drug/implant-related problems
Hypotony	Steroid-induced cataract
Vitreous hemorrhage	Intraocular pressure elevation
Infectious endophthalmitis	Glaucoma
Traumatic cataract	Cytomegalovirus retinitis
Retinal tear	Vitreous band formation with or without macular traction
Retinal detachment	Impaired glucose tolerance
Subconjunctival hemorrhage	Drug cylinder breakdown or detachment
Implantation wound site infection	

treatment of severe cases of noninfectious intermediate uveitis, posterior uveitis, or panuveitis. Of note, clinical trials for Retisert® were previously started but later abandoned for the indications of diabetic macular edema and exudative AMD.

Other slow-release corticosteroid intravitreal implants, including biodegradable ones, are also under development with the hope that they will have similar efficacy to the Retisert® implant, but with fewer adverse effects.

Overall, the benefit and effectiveness of local administration of corticosteroids (injections or intravitreal implant) for use in posterior uveitis has not been clearly demonstrated over the long term, while there is a long list of adverse ocular effects that threaten sight for iatrogenic reasons. In addition, the use of these agents in most cases is limited since PSII and STOI are frequently bilateral and local applications have been targeted toward patients with uniocular disease. Therefore, as a general rule, this treatment modality should always be used in conjunction with proper immunomodulatory therapy in anything other than mild PSII (see chap. 4).

PERIOPERATIVE MEDICAL MANAGEMENT

Although once believed too dangerous to consider, surgical techniques have advanced to the point today where most procedures can be performed safely in eyes with intraocular inflammation that is more or less quiescent. In particular, the use of small incisions in cataract surgery and 23- or 25-gauge instruments in vitrectomy have greatly lessened surgical trauma to the eye and therefore lessened both the degree of postoperative inflammation and the risk of disease recurrence. There are, however, a few important points to consider with regards to the perioperative medical management of uveitic eyes undergoing surgery as discussed below. Specifics on surgical techniques are not covered here, as they are extensively described in other reference books that the reader is also encouraged to consult.

Preoperative Anti-inflammatory Therapy

The general rule of thumb is to advance treatment to the point where the eye is quiescent for at least three months prior to surgery, that is, less than 1+ cells (at very most) in the anterior chamber and no posterior inflammatory attacks. However, there are instances of STOI in which a surgical intervention *is* the treatment required in order to prevent irreversible visual loss, for example, as in an eye with intractable glaucoma requiring filtering surgery. In these more desperate cases, one cannot wait for all inflammation to disappear before surgery and one may be forced to operate on an actively inflamed eye. Likewise, a dense cataract may interfere with appropriate monitoring of the fundus, and again force one's hand to perform surgery.

One method commonly used to enhance surgical success is to increase the preoperative medical regimen even in a quiet eye. In the case of anterior segment surgery, such as cataract or glaucoma, an increase in topical corticosteroids may be adequate (e.g., betamethasone or prednisone drops 4–6 times a day). In the case of posterior segment surgery, uveitis specialists in the past have often utilized a short course of oral corticosteroids (e.g., 20–30 mg/day prednisolone), starting perhaps one week prior to surgery and then continuing for two to three weeks after surgery, with or without a taper depending on the disease process. An alternative strategy is to increase the immunosuppressive regimen for a few months before and after surgery. However, a posterior sub-Tenon's injection of corticosteroid at the time of surgery (see below) will generally obviate the need for an increase in the systemic medical regimen for many patients. Some surgeons adopt a more aggressive approach, namely, to ensure that the eye is as quiet as possible during the immediate two weeks prior to surgery and then to administer perioperative IV methylprednisolone for three days (one day before, on the day of, and one day after surgery). Additional intensive postoperative topical or oral therapy is then given as indicated by the degree of inflammation in the postoperative period.

Intraoperative Anti-inflammatory Therapy

As stated above, a posterior sub-Tenon's injection, usually of triamcinolone acetonide, may be given at the conclusion of surgery in the operating room. This is particularly effective in treating existing CME or preventing postoperative CME. The conjunctiva is already opened in the course of surgery, and therefore insertion of a needle or the blunt 23-gauge, curved cannula is a simple adjunctive procedure to perform, with a "depot" anti-inflammatory effect that will last for two to three months. The dose given is the same as for this type of injection in the clinic, i.e., 20 to 40 mg in 0.5 to 1.0 cc. Alternatively, some surgeons will elect to give an intravitreal injection of 4 mg in 0.1 cc of triamcinolone acetonide instead, although in a vitrectomized eye the half-life of the drug will be shortened with a corresponding decrease in the duration of anti-inflammatory efficacy. Of course, when giving such corticosteroid injections, it is ideal if the eye is already pseudophakic or is undergoing cataract removal at the time of surgery. Of note, there is rarely a rise in IOP observed in relation to local corticosteroid injections given intraoperatively, most likely due to the overall decrease in ciliary body function immediately after surgery.

The option of giving pulse IV methylprednisolone may be considered for high-risk patients (67). However, one study found that one dose of IV methylprednisolone (15 mg/kg) administered 30 minutes before surgery was inferior to a two week preoperative course of oral prednisolone (0.5 mg/kg/day) followed by a postoperative taper (68). The choice of delivery (periocular injection, intravitreal injection, or intravenous administration) of intraoperative corticosteroids must in the end be tailored to the particular diagnosis, condition of the eye, and the medical status of the patient.

Given the variety (even if systematic) of approaches in most uveitis services, consensus is currently hard to achieve. We therefore have generated a system for guidance, where choice of regime depends on the severity of previously treated uveitis, the degree of surgical manipulation required, and level of current immunosuppression (Box 3).

Since a subconjunctival injection of corticosteroid at the end of surgery will aid in reducing postoperative inflammation in the anterior segment, this should be routinely performed for most eyes (also refer to chap. 4). This is particularly imperative in patients with a history of severe anterior segment inflammation and/or iris synechia formation.

Box 3 Treatment Regimens for Surgery

Patient on immunosuppression	Patient not on immunosuppression	
Previous STOI or high-risk surgery	**Low-risk surgery**	**High-risk surgery**
Preoperative corticosteroid increase	Sub-Tenon's triamcinolone	IV Methylprednisolone (500 mg)
IV Methylprednisolone (500 mg)	Hourly topical corticosteroids	Sub-Tenon's triamcinolone
Postoperative reducing corticosteroids		Hourly topical corticosteroids
Sub-Tenon's triamcinolone		

For all cases one may consider the use of depot intravitreal triamcinolone

Postoperative Anti-inflammatory Therapy

The major complications after surgery particular to an eye with a history of intraocular inflammation are hypotony, posterior iris synechia, pupillary membrane formation, posterior capsular opacification, CME, secondary epiretinal membrane formation, and disease recurrence or worsening. The hope is that with appropriate pre- and perioperative immunosuppression, the risk of these complications developing can be prevented and further reduced by the aggressive use of local corticosteroid administration. If an eye has a history of severe anterior segment inflammation, especially in the presence of iris synechia, anterior segment complications may be reduced by the use of frequent administration of topical corticosteroids, up to once an hour if necessary, for the first one to two weeks. For an eye with a history of posterior segment inflammation, the placement of a posterior sub-Tenon's corticosteroid injection at the time of surgery is usually effective in suppressing postoperative inflammation for the first two to three months (Box 3). However, thereafter, one may observe development of macular edema, which would then have to be addressed with a repeat posterior sub-Tenon's injection or other treatment modalities as if one were treating PSII and, particularly, STOI (see chap. 4).

SUMMARY

The treatment of PSII may appear to be a daunting and potentially dangerous task to the ophthalmologist. Alliance with appropriate internal medicine specialists is strongly encouraged, and continuing "education" of the patient in terms of risks and benefits of treatment is essential. In cases of sight-threatening ocular inflammation, one should not hesitate to treat, since early action may be imperative to preserving useful vision. Until recently, such action has generally consisted of the use of systemic corticosteroids first, followed by the addition of or conversion to immunosuppressive agents. However, with the advent of biologic therapy, we now have the ability to more specifically modulate the immune system in order to control inflammation and possibly induce remission.

REFERENCES

1. Oldenburg B, Hommes D. Biological therapies in inflammatory bowel disease: top-down or bottom-up? Curr Opin Gastroenterol 2007; 23:395–399.
2. Hommes D, Baert F, Van Assche G, et al. Management of recent onset Crohn's disease: a controlled, randomized trial comparing step-up and top-down therapy. Gastroenterology 2005; 129:371.

3. Jabs DA, Rosenbaum JT, Foster CS, et al. Guidelines for the use of immunosuppressive drugs in patients with ocular inflammatory disorders: recommendations of an expert panel. Am J Ophthalmol 2000; 130:492–513.

4. Read RW, Yu F, Accorinti M, et al. Evaluation of the effect on outcomes of the route of administration of corticosteroids in acute Vogt-Koyanagi-Harada disease. Am J Ophthalmol 2006; 142:119–124.

5. Okada AA. Immunomodulatory therapy for ocular inflammatory disease: a basic manual and review of the literature. Ocular Immunol Inflamm 2005; 13:335–351.

6. Yazici H, Pazarli H, Barnes CG, et al. A controlled trial of azathioprine in Behçet's syndrome. N Engl J Med 1990; 322:281–285.

7. Singh G, Fries JF, Spitz P, Williams CA. Toxic effects of azathioprine in rheumatoid arthritis. A national post-marketing perspective. Arthritis Rheum 1989; 32:837–843.

8. Kump LI, Castaneda RA, Androudi SN, et al. Visual outcomes in children with juvenile idiopathic arthritis-associated uveitis. Ophthalmology 2006; 113: 1874–1877.

9. Weinblatt ME. Toxicity of low dose methotrexate in rheumatoid arthritis. J Rheumatol 1985; 12:35–39.

10. Thorne JE, Jabs DA, Qazi FA, et al. Mycophenolate mofetil therapy for inflammatory eye disease. Ophthalmology 2005; 112:1472–1477.

11. Mok CC, Lau CS, Wong RW. Risk factors for ovarian failure in patients with systemic lupus erythematosus receiving cyclophsophamide therapy. Arthritis Rheum 1998; 41:831–837.

12. Fukutani K, Ishida H, Shinohara M, et al. Suppression of spermatogenesis in patients with Behçet's disease treated with cyclophophamide and colchicine. Fertil Steril 1981; 36:76–80.

13. Rosenbaum JT. Treatment of severe refractory uveitis with intravenous cyclophosphamide. J Rheumatol 1994; 21:123–125.

14. Ozyazgan Y, Yurdakul S, Yazici H, et al. Low dose cyclosporine A versus pulsed cyclophosphamide in Behçet's syndrome: a single masked trial. Br J Ophthalmol 1992; 76:241–243.

15. Ando K, Fujino Y, Hijikata K, et al. Epidemiological features and visual prognosis of Behçet's disease. Jpn J Ophthalmol 1999; 43:312–317.

16. Talar-Williams C, Hijazi YM, Walther MM, et al. Cyclophosphamide-induced cystitis and bladder cancer in patients with Wegener granulomatosis. Ann Intern Med 1996; 124:477–484.

17. BenEzra D, Cohen E, Chajek T, et al. Evaluation of conventional therapy versus cyclosporine A in Behçet's syndrome. Transplant Proc 1988; 20:136–143.

18. Masuda K, Nakajima A, Urayama A, et al. Double-masked trial of cyclosporine versus colchicine and long-term open study of cyclosporine in Behçet's disease. Lancet 1989; 1(8647):1093–1096.

19. Rodriguez F, Krayenbuhl JC, Harrison WB, et al. Renal biopsy findings and followup of renal function in rheumatoid arthritis patients treated with cyclosporine A. An update from the International Kidney Biopsy Registry. Arthritis Rheum 1996; 39:1491–1498.

20. Kotter I, Gunaydin I, Batra M, et al. CNS involvement occurs more frequently in patients with Behçet's disease under cyclosporin A (CSA) than under other medications—results of a retrospective analysis of 117 cases. Clin Rheumatol 2005; 25:482–486.

21. Murphy CC, Greiner K, Plskova J, et al. Cyclosporin versus tacrolimus therapy for posterior and intermediate uveitis. Arch Ophthalmol 2005; 123:634–641.

22. Ligtenberg G, Hene RJ, Blankestijn PJ, et al. Cardiovascular risk factors in renal transplant patients: cyclosporin A versus tacrolimus. J Am Soc Nephrol 2001; 12:368–373.

23. Hogan AC, McAvoy CE, Dick AD, et al. Long-term efficacy and tolerance of tacrolimus for the treatment of uveitis. Ophthalmology 2007; 114:1000–1006.

24. Imrie FR, Dick AD. Biologics in the treatment of uveitis. Curr Opin Ophthalmol 2007; 18:481–486.

25. Durand JM, Kaplanski G, Telle H, et al. Beneficial effects of interferon-α2b in Behçet's disease. Arthritis Rheum 1993; 36:1025–1026.

26. Feron EJ, Rothova A, van Hagen PM, et al. Interferon-α2b for refractory ocular Behçet's disease. Lancet 1994; 343:1428(letter).

27. Kotter I, Zierhut M, Eckstein AK, et al. Human recombinant interferon alfa-2a for the treatment of Behçet's disease with sight threatening posterior or panuveitis. Br J Ophthalmol 2003; 87:423–431.

28. Tugal-Tutkun I, Guney-Tefekli E, Urgancioglu M. Results of interferon-alfa therapy in patients with Behcet uveitis. Graefes Arch Clin Exp Ophthalmol 2006; 244:1692–1695.

29. Bodaghi B, Gendron G, Wechsler B, et al. Efficacy of interferon alpha in the treatment of refractory and sight threatening uveitis: a retrospective monocentric study of 45 patients. Br J Ophthlamol 2007; 91:335–339.

30. Plskova J, Greiner K, Forrester JV. Interferon alpha as an effective treatment for noninfectious posterior uveitis and panuveitis. Am J Ophthalmol 2007; 144:55–61.

31. Plskova J, Greiner K, Muckersie E, et al. Interferon-alpha: a key factor in automimmune disease? Invest Ophthalmol Vis Sci 2006; 47:3946–3950.

32. Maini R, St. Clair WE, Breedveld F, et al. Infliximab (chimeric anti-tumour necorsis factor a monoclonal antibody) versus placebo in rheumatoid arthritis patients receiving concomitant methotrexate: a randomized phase III trial. Lancet 1999; 354:1932–1939.

33. Sands BE, Anderson FH, Bernstein CN, et al. Infliximab maintenance therapy for fistulizing Crohn's disease. N Engl J Med 2004; 350:876–885.

34. Braun J, de Keyser F, Brandt J, et al. New treatment options in spondyloarthro-pathies: increasing evidence for significant efficacy of anti-tumor necrosis factor therapy. Curr Opin Rheumatol 2001; 13:245–249.

35. Suhler EB, Smith JR, Wertheim MS, et al. A prospective trial of infliximab therapy for refractory uveitis: preliminary safety and efficacy outcomes. Arch Ophthalmol 2005; 123:903–912.

36. Lindstedt EW, Baarsma GS, Kuijpers RWAM, et al. Anti-TNF-α therapy for sight threatening uveitis. Br J Ophthalmol 2005; 89:533–536.

37. Sobrin L, Kim EC, Christen W, et al. Infliximab therapy for the treatment of refractory ocular inflammatory disease. Arch Ophthalmol 2007; 125:895–900.

38. Ohno S, Nakamura S, Hori S, et al. Efficacy, safety, and pharmacokinetics of multiple administration of infliximab in Behçet's disease with refractory uveor-etinitis. J Rheumatol 2004; 31:1362–1368.

39. Tugal-Tutkun I, Mudun A, Urgancioglu M, et al. Efficacy of infliximab in the treatment of uveitis that is resistant to treatment with the combination of azathioprine, cyclosporine, and corticosteroids in Behçet's disease. Arthritis Rheum 2005; 52:2478–2484.

40. Abu El-Asrar AM, Abboud EB, Aldibhi H, et al. Long-term safety and efficacy of infliximab therapy in refractory uveitis due to Behçet's disease. Int Ophthalmol 2005; 26:83–92.

41. Jabs DA, Nussenblatt RB, Rosenbaum JT. Standardization of Uveitis Nomenclature (SUN) Working Group. Standardization of uveitis nomenclature for reporting clinical data. Results of the first international workshop. Am J Ophthalmol 2005; 140:509–516.

42. Hochberg MC, Lebwohl MG, Plevy SE, et al. The benefit/risk profile of TNF-blocking agents: findings of a consensus panel. Semin Arthritis Rheum 2005; 34:819–836.

43. Rosenbaum JT. Blind insight: eyeing anti-tumor necrosis factor treatment in uveitis associated with Behçet's disease. 2004; 31:1241–1243.

44. Vermeire S, Noman M, Assche GV, et al. Effectiveness of concomitant immunosuppressive therapy in suppressing the formation of antibodies to infliximab in Crohn's disease. Gut 2007; 56:1226–1231.

45. Scott DL, Kingsley GH. Tumor necrosis factor inhibitors for rheumatoid arthritis. N Engl J Med 2006; 355:704–712.

46. Reiff A, Takei S, Sadeghi S, et al. Etanercept therapy in children with treatment-resistant uveitis. Arthritis Rheum 2001; 44:1411–1415.

47. Mushtaq B, Saeed T, Situnayake RD, Murray PI. Adalimumab for sight-threatening uveitis in Behçet's disease. Eye 2007; 21:824–825.

48. Biester S, Deuter C, Michels H, et al. Adalimumab in the therapy of uveitis in childhood. Br J Ophthalmol 2007; 91:319–324.

49. Lockwood CM, Hale G, Waldman H, et al. Remission induction in Behçet's disease following lymphocyte depletion by the anti-CD52 antibody CAMPATH–1H. Rheumatology 2003; 42:1539–1544.

50. Dick AD, Meyer P, James T, et al. CAMPATH-1H therapy for the treatment of refractory ocular inflammatory disease. Br J Ophthalmol 2000; 84:107–109.

51. Nussenblatt RB, Peterson JS, Foster CS, et al. Initial evaluation of subcutaneous daclizumab treatments for noninfectious uveitis: a multicenter noncomparative interventional case series. Ophthalmology 2005; 112:764–770.

52. Teoh SCB, Sharma S, Hogan A, et al. Tailoring biologic therapy: anakinra treatment of CINCA-associated posterior uveitis. Br J Ophthalmol 2007; 91:263–267.

53. Okada AA, Wakabayashi T, Morimura Y, et al. Trans-Tenon's retrobulbar triamcinolone infusion for the treatment of uveitis. Br J Ophthalmol 2003; 87:968–971.

54. Danis RP, Ciulla TA, Pratt LM, et al. Intravitreal triamcinolone acetonide in exudative age-related macular degeneration. Retina 2000; 20:244–250.

55. Young S, Larkin G, Branley M, et al. Safety and efficacy of intravitreal triamcinolone for cystoid macular oedema in uveitis. Clin Exp Ophthalmol 2001; 29:2–6.

56. Antcliff RJ, Spalton DJ, Stanford MR, et al. Intravitreal triamcinolone for uveitic cystoid macular edema: an optical coherence tomography study. Ophthalmology 2001; 108:765–772.

57. Martidis A, Duker JS, Puliafito CA. Intravitreal triamcinolone for refractory cystoid macular edema secondary to birdshot retinochoroidopathy. Arch Ophthalmol 2001; 119:1380–1383.

58. McCuen BW, Bessler M, Tano Y, et al. The lack of toxicity of intravitreally administered triamcinolone acetonide. Am J Ophthlamol 1981; 91:785–788.

59. Sutter FK, Gillies MC. Pseudo-endophthalmitis after intravitreal injection of triamcinolone. Br J Ophthalmol 2003; 87:972–974.

60. Enaida H, Hata Y, Ueno A, et al. Possible benefits of triamcinolone-assisted pars plana vitrectomy for retinal diseases. Retina 2003; 23:764–770.

61. Mosfeghi DM, Kaiser PM, Scott IU, et al. Acute endophthalmitis following intravitreal triamcinolone acetonide injection. Am J Ophthalmol 2003; 136:791–796.

62. Gillies MC, Simpson JM, Billson FA, et al. Safety of an intravitreal injection of triamcinolone: results from a randomized clinical trial. Arch Ophthalmol 2004; 122:336–340.

63. Jaffe GJ, Martin D, Callanan D, et al. Fluocinolone acetonide implant (Retisert) for noninfectious posterior uveitis: thirty-four-week results of a multicenter randomized clinical study. Ophthalmology 2006; 113:1020–1027.

64. Goldstein DA, Godfrey DG, Hall A, et al. Intraocular pressure in patients with uveitis treated with fluocinolone acetonide implants. Arch Ophthalmol 2007; 125:1478–1485.

65. Ufret-Vincenty RL, Singh RP, Lowder CY, et al. Cytomegalovirus retinitis after fluocinolone acetonide (Retisert™) implant. Am J Ophthalmol 2007; 143:334–335.

66. Galor A, Margolis R, Kaiser PK, et al. Vitreous band formation and the sustained-release intravitreal fluocinolone (Retisert) implant. Arch Opthalmol 2007; 125: 836–838.

67. Okhravi N, Lightman SL, Towler HMA. Assessment of visual outcome after cataract surgery in patients with uveitis. Ophthalmology 1999; 106:710–722.

68. Meacock WR, Spalton DJ, Bender L, et al. Steroid prophylaxis in eyes with uveitis undergoing phacoemulsification. Br J Ophthalmol 2004; 88:1122–1124.

6
Research Questions

INTRODUCTION

As reiterated a number of times in this handbook, ocular inflammation, particularly sight-threatening uveitis, strikes a feeling of defeat in many ophthalmologists, and they gladly search around for a "uveitis specialist" who will take responsibility for the patient's treatment and especially relieve him/her of the risk of either misdiagnosing the condition (e.g., missing an intraocular lymphoma) or shortening the patient's life by administration of some toxic drug regime. More unsettling than anything is the feeling of not truly understanding what is going on as the patient loses vision. This chapter aims to dispel a few of the uncertainties and to pinpoint areas where research in the future might be directed to allow us to achieve a higher level of understanding of the condition and developing better, more targeted therapies.

THE CLINICAL PROBLEM

The patient with sight-threatening ocular inflammation (STOI) presents more than one clinical problem.

Diagnosis

Ocular inflammation (uveitis) does not rank high on the list of recognized major causes of blindness. One of the reasons for this is the lack of a unifying classification for the many diseases that are included in this category of disorders. The bewildering range of diagnoses, the many causes of both infectious and noninfectious STOI, and the difficulty in defining what constitutes a threat to vision, all contribute to this clinical problem. Each individually may be a rare presentation, but when all causes are combined, "uveitis" remains a significant cause of blindness worldwide and certainly in developed countries, within the working age population.

In this handbook, we have attempted to bring some degree of order to this confusion. While the specific diagnosis is important, particularly when wishing to provide a visual prognosis in any individual patient, when it is reduced to its essential elements, ocular inflammation only asks two central questions: is the disease infectious or not and what is the risk of visual loss? In this context, a precise diagnosis may not be as important as assessing the degree of inflammation. Furthermore, it is important, if only to highlight the size of the problem to epidemiologists and public health authorities, that much of this visual disability is avoidable with correct and safe management. In this regard, therefore, it is also important that uveitis specialists come together with a uniform grading system for disease (i.e., ocular inflammation generally) activity, and the Standardization of Uveitis Nomenclature (SUN) grading system (1) is a significant step forward in developing a standardized grading system for evaluating the severity of inflammation.

However, the two questions outlined above do raise two important areas for further research: (*i*) How can we improve our diagnostic ability to exclude infectious disease? (*ii*) Do we have better ways of assessing the threat to vision?

Investigative Tools

Excluding infectious disease is notoriously difficult and many suspected cases go undetected or only become accurately diagnosed when they respond to a therapeutic trial, e.g., in cases of peripheral retinal vasculitis due to tuberculosis. In addition, the amplifying effect of intercurrent infection, in patients who undergo a recrudescence temporally linked to the infection, points significantly toward a role for innate immune mechanisms triggering an attack of uveitis (see chap. 1). While experimental models are useful in revealing mechanisms whereby this might occur, the clinical problem of knowing what emphasis to place on such mechanisms remains a challenge. The possibility that more sensitive biomarkers will identify nonspecific inflammatory mechanisms (or even specific infectious agents) may be worthy of exploration. Development of a greater range of specific "primers" for detection of specific organisms by polymerase chain reaction (PCR) will improve diagnosis. In the meantime, research tools such as flow cytometry have revealed the value of using "activation markers" on circulating blood cells and cells from ocular samples to monitor

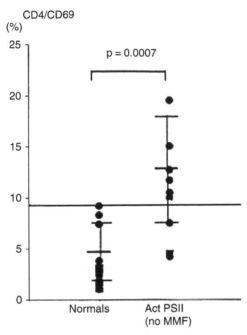

CD4/CD69
(%)

Figure 1 Peripheral blood CD4$^+$ T-cell CD69 expression (unstimulated) in control groups not receiving MMF therapy. Patients not receiving MMF therapy with active PSII [act PSII (no MMF), $n = 10$] were compared with healthy volunteers (normals, $n = 21$). Levels shown are mean percentages ±SD of CD69 expression on CD3$^+$CD4$^+$ cells, with comparison made (*horizontal line*) for both control groups with 95% (mean ±2SD) of the normal range. *Abbreviations*: MMF, mycophenolate mofetil; PSII, posterior segment intraocular inflammation. *Source*: From Ref. 2.

response to therapy (2) as well as to further highlight pathogenic mechanisms (Fig. 1) (3–5). It is envisaged that gene chip and proteome-based microarray technology might ultimately provide customized diagnostic and therapeutic tools, akin to the developments being made in lymphoproliferative diseases.

The second question of developing better ways of assessing the threat to vision is also under intensive scrutiny with new imaging and functional modalities. For instance, the new high-resolution ocular coherence tomography (OCT) machines almost provide in vivo "histological sections" of the retina (Fig. 2) and this combined with novel adaptive optics technology and electrophysiological and visual field functional analyses will allow us even more sensitive modalities for evaluation of our patients. A logistic constraint on these optical imaging modalities is the presence of vitreous opacities; however, improvements in ultrasound technology including ultrasonic biomicroscopy are providing important and useful information although these are still not applicable in any major way to evaluation of the central posterior segment at present.

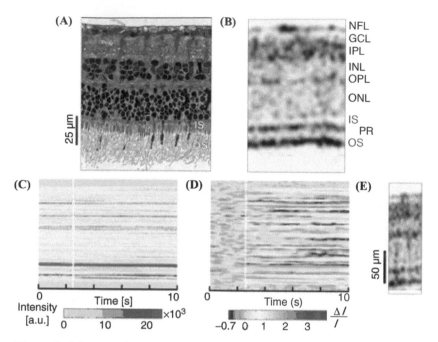

Figure 2 Morphological and functional retinal imaging with UHROCT. Comparison between a histological cross section (**A**); an OCT morphological tomogram (**B**) of the isolated retina demonstrates the ability of UHROCT to visualize the layered retinal structure. OCT M-scan (**C**; optical signal measured at one position over time) and differential M-scan (**D**; produced from **C** by subtracting the background signal, calculated as a time average of the preactivation depth scans from the entire M-scan) are compared with a morphological UHROCT tomogram (**E**) of the location where the OCT M-scan was acquired. The white strips mark the onset and duration of the white light flash. *Abbreviations*: UHROCT, ultrahigh resolution ocular coherence tomography; NFL, nerve fiber layer; GCL, ganglion cell layer; IPL, inner plexiform layer; INL, inner nuclear layer; OPL, outer plexiform layer; ONL, outer nuclear layer; IS, inner segment; PR, photo receptors; OS, outer segment. *Source*: From Ref. 22.

Treatment

We have come a long way since cyclosporine was introduced in the mid 1980s for the control of STOI (6). As detailed in chapters 4 and 5, we now have many new drugs which allow us to avoid the many, severely debilitating side effects of systemic steroids. Steroids remain an important drug in the control of ocular inflammation, but usually in low dose and in combination with other immunosuppressants.

However, the side effects of the newer immunosuppressants are serious and can be debilitating, even, on rare occasions, life threatening, as well as having significant effects on overall quality of life. The patient, after informed discussion, has a difficult decision to make balancing the preservation of his vision with the overall effects on his lifestyle and his survival.

The new generation of drugs, including the biologics, has brought new hope to patients with STOI (as well as many other immune-mediated and autoimmune diseases). However, they are extremely expensive, require individualized administration protocols depending on the drug, and in practice are available to only a very small number of patients with ocular inflammation even in privileged western countries. From a research perspective, many other issues arise; for instance, although we know a great deal about the mechanism of action of these drugs, we are learning continuously. For example, it was initially believed that the calcineurin-inhibitor cyclosporine (and tacrolimus) functioned by inhibiting interleukin (IL)-2, a growth factor required for T-cell function. However, recent studies have shown that cyclosporin inhibits transforming growth factor-β (TGF-β) (7), a cytokine known to be an inhibitor of immune responses when acting in isolation, but now recognized as an inducer of IL-17$^+$ Th17 cells when acting in synergy with IL-6 (7). IL-17$^+$ T cells are important in defense against infectious agents but are also involved in some T-cell autoimmune-mediated diseases including uveitis (see chap. 1).

This raises the question about what are we targeting in our treatment of autoimmune uveitis and indeed autoimmunity generally. In fact, what exactly is our therapeutic strategy? This depends critically on what we understand about the pathogenesis of the disease and for this we have to rely on animal models since they provide us with the opportunity to investigate the initial stages of the disease. When information derived from these studies is combined with information derived from research on clinical samples from patients (mostly nonocular samples), the prospect of designing intelligence-based treatment modalities customized for individual patients arises.

UNDERSTANDING PATHOGENESIS— THE USE OF ANIMAL MODELS

Models of Uveitis-Uveoretinitis

Research into uveitis has been dogged by false trails from the beginning. Since many cases of uveitis could not be designated "infectious," it was assumed that the disease was predominantly autoimmune or at least autoinflammatory in nature. Since the uveal tract was the apparent site of the inflammation, it was also assumed that the target autoantigen resided in the uveal tract. After many years of trying to induce experimental uveitis using extracts of uveal tissue in an emulsion of mycobacterial "adjuvant" (the standard method of inducing experimental autoimmune diseases with the immunologists "dirty little secret" as Janeway described it), it was found by Waldon Wacker that the retina contained the most potent autoantigen (8). The first retinal antigen, soluble or retinal S-antigen generated a great flurry of activity in the search, first for autoantibodies and then for antigen-specific cellular responses to retinal antigens in humans. However, as the models progressed from guinea pigs to rats to primates and mice, it was realized that there is a plethora of retinal antigens, all of which can produce experimental uveitis varying on a basic pathological theme. Indeed, even a single antigen can reproduce many of the clinical and histological findings or a range of human disorders depending on the dose of antigen, the species and model, the route of administration, and the immunocompetent status of the animal (9). This is not to say that certain forms of uveitis, particularly posterior uveitis, are more likely to be due to a specific antigen; for example, Vogt-Koyanagi-Harada's disease seems to be a form of autoimmunity to melanin-associated antigens, particularly tyrosinase-related peptides (Trp1 and Trp2) (10). In addition, there are certain forms of experimental uveitis that are restricted to the anterior segment, and even some in which endotoxin produces a self-limiting predominantly anterior uveitis. Attempts to induce human-specific models have also been tried using transgenic mice in which human major histocompatibility complex (MHC) class II or class I molecules have been expressed. Finally, a spontaneous model of uveoretinitis has recently been described using a double transgenic model in which a foreign antigen is expressed in the retina under the control of the retina-specific antigen, interphotoreceptor retinal-binding protein (11). These models are very useful since they allow study of many aspects of the disease (see box 1).

Box 1
What do animal models tell us about?
- Disease mechanisms from the initiation of the disease to the effector mechanisms
- The role of specific target antigens in the eye
- The relative importance of different cells in inducing and regulating the disease
- The contribution of innate (nonspecific) versus adaptive immune mechanisms to pathogenesis
- Development of novel treatments
- Fundamental studies of tolerance mechanisms (autoimmunity generally)

Do the Animal Models Faithfully Represent the Clinical Disease?

Central to the use of animal models is how faithfully they represent the clinical disease. There is a considerable spectrum of clinical uveitis presentations from acute aggressive retinal vasculitis with panuveitis and hypopyon (as in severe Behçet's disease) to low-grade subretinal inflammatory neovascular membranes occurring in the absence of significant associated inflammation (as in some of the white dot syndromes). Immunization of mice with retinal antigens in adjuvant (as stated above) can induce similar models, and with newer imaging techniques, an excellent clinicopathological correlation can be made.

What Have We Learned from the Animal Models?

The flood of information from the animal models has been continuous and expanding: for instance we know from these models that STOI is a cell-mediated disease, originally considered to be CD4 Th1 cell driven but recently shown to occur as subtypes, depending on Th17, Th1, and Th2 predominance (see chap. 1). The role of antibodies and B cells has been less clear, but certainly in some uveitis variants are probably significant (12), and complement seems to play a role in severe disease. These models lend themselves to in vivo imaging so that cellular trafficking and interactions can be modeled directly, and the role of specific molecules such as CD44 and P-selectin glycoprotein ligand-1 in directing pathogenic cells to sites of disease in the retina has been shown. These studies are of direct relevance to blocking therapies since they open up potential therapeutic approaches using monoclonal antibodies (biologics, see chap. 5) to control inflammation (see also next section). The example par excellence of this approach is the introduction of anti–tumor necrosis factor-α (anti-TNF-α) therapy for intractable uveitis, but the approach goes back many years. Cyclosporine A was first used in experimental uveitis before being introduced to the clinic. Many new potential therapeutic approaches are possible as a result of these studies.

Animal models have revealed some fundamental aspects of the regulation of autoimmune disease. For instance, the identification of the autoimmune regulator (AIRE) gene has shown how a single gene in the thymus can exert control over multiple organ-specific autoimmune diseases including uveoretinitis, and furthermore that lack of expression of a single autoantigen in the thymus is sufficient to trigger autoimmune retinopathy even in the presence of the AIRE gene (13). This has major significance for mechanisms of tolerance, and indeed bystander tolerance mechanisms in general, and how this process actually works is a major question for immunologists.

The wide range of retinal antigens which can induce disease has also led us to rethink our approach to the diagnosis, investigation, and treatment of autoimmune uveoretinitis. For instance, the notion of "antigen specificity" has receded when it became clear that there was no good correlation between specific autoantibodies or cell-specific responses and levels of activity, that these immunological responses occurred in a large proportion of normal individuals, and in any case, when animals developed autoimmune inflammation in response to one antigen, there was spread of autoreactivity to other antigens in what became termed "epitope spreading." This is part of the overall notion of "bystander damage," the corollary to "bystander tolerance" mentioned above.

As a result, work on the animal models has also redirected our thinking regarding how to approach management of autoimmune disease, with greater emphasis on controlling effector mechanisms of tissue damage. After all, most patients who present with STOI have already had the disease for some time; if they are infectious, they may also have an immune component to the disease as in tuberculosis in which there is an immune response to mycobacterial antigen as well as unchecked proliferation of the infective organism. If they have a viral illness, they may actually be experiencing a measure of immune evasion, or even suppression, which is contributing to the disease. If the disease is auto-inflammatory, although it may have been triggered by exposure to some infectious agent, in the presence of ongoing STOI, the patient is more likely to be responding to more than one retinal autoantigen released during tissue inflam-mation and antigen-specific therapy may be less effective (although see comments on the AIRE gene above). Currently, therefore, many experimental physicians are looking at ways of limiting tissue damage by inhibiting effector T cells or their cytokine and chemokine effector molecules.

NOVEL THERAPIES

In the face of the mechanistic complexity of autoimmune disease in which there is breakdown in tolerance to self-antigens (mostly retinal antigens in the case of uveitis), several novel approaches are being explored to attempt to restore tolerance. These include gene therapy, small inhibitory RNA (siRNA) (gene knockdown) therapy, and dendritic cell vaccination via induction of T regulatory cells (Tregs).

Gene Therapy

Gene therapy using adenovirus (AV or AAV) vectors delivered into the subretinal space has been trialed in experimental models of retinal degeneration, and initial steps have been taken toward full-scale clinical trials in humans. Similar approaches have been proposed for regulation of ocular inflammation, and some early experimental studies have been undertaken using vectors expressing IL-10 (an immunosuppressive cytokine) (14). Another study has demonstrated that plasmid expression of a soluble chimeric human TNF-α receptor protein (thereby blocking the effects of TNF-α) can have a marked inhibitory effect when the vector is delivered to the ciliary body via electrotransfer (15). Thus the potential for gene therapy in uveoretinitis shows promise for the future provided the correct targets are identified, and that the vectors themselves allow sustained effects at least for the duration of a potentially chronic disease, without causing toxic effects.

Gene Knockdown

An alternative to delivering agents that incorporate themselves into the cells of the eye and synthesize potentially anti-inflammatory molecules is to introduce molecules which inhibit the synthesis of proinflammatory molecules. The discovery of siRNA molecules, which act by blocking the synthesis of proteins by binding to relevant complementary sequences in the gene of interest, offers a new and exciting technology to downregulate inflammatory processes. siRNA has been shown to work very effectively, and specifically in vitro, but the evidence for in vivo effects has been more difficult to reproduce. No such approach has been tried yet in experimental uveoretinitis but it is only a matter of time. In vivo effects have been demonstrated in other systems such as experimental autoimmune encephalomyelitis (animal model for multiple sclerosis) (16).

Dendritic Cell Vaccination and Induction of Tregs

Dendritic cells (DC) are classically considered to be the most potent antigen-presenting cells in the organism and indeed this is one of their roles, namely the induction of adaptive immune responses to foreign antigens. However, in the resting state it has been realized that the major function of DC is to promote and maintain tolerance to self-antigens (tolerizing DC). This they do by patrolling the tissues, capturing shed self-antigens from cells in the process of normal metabolic functions and transporting them to draining lymph nodes where they present the antigen to T cells and promote tolerance. In fact, the draining lymph node in the resting physiological state has been described as an immune-privileged organ similar to the original description of the eye itself.

Immune privilege is thus a form of tolerance and is induced in part by induction of a special set of T cells known as regulatory cells (or Tregs) (see chap. 1). There are several types of Tregs; one type comprises around 5% to 10% of the CD4$^+$ T cells pool, expresses special markers such as high levels of CD25 and the Treg-specific transcription factor FoxP3, and appears to exert its regulatory effect though the immunoinhibitory cytokine TGF-β. CD4$^+$CD25$^+$

Tregs can be induced by tolerizing DC and indeed this is the main mechanism thought to underlie mucosal tolerance. In this process, antigen administered via the nasal or gut mucosa is picked up by DC in the lining mucosal tissues and transported to the draining lymph nodes where they induce Tregs. This type of induced "mucosal tolerance" has been shown to prevent induction of many experimental autoimmune diseases including experimental autoimmune uveoretinitis and has been tested in clinical trails of multiple sclerosis and uveitis, with a small clinical benefit. The main problem with this approach has been the lack of strength of the overall tolerance response.

Other strategies have therefore been investigated: one of these is to attempt to induce a high concentration of antigen-specific Tregs by administering "tolerizing DC" loaded with specific antigen. The key to this is to generate sufficient numbers of tolerizing DC, itself a difficult cell to define, since DC demonstrate considerable plasticity and there is a fine line between inducing tolerance or immunity. Indeed DC vaccination is mostly being studied from the standpoint of stimulating immune responses, e.g., to tumors as in cancer immunotherapy or infectious disease. Tolerizing DC can be generated in vitro from bone marrow or circulating DC precursors if the conditions are correct. Thus, antigen-loaded DC have been shown to prevent many experimental autoimmune diseases and most recently to prevent ongoing autoimmune diabetes in a transgenic mouse model. Tolerizing DC have also been shown to prevent experimental autoimmune uveoretinitis (17,18) and this they do via expanding the population of antigen-specific Tregs in the draining lymph node.

The exciting prospect is therefore presented in which it would be possible to regulate a patient's STOI by culturing autologous DC from the blood in the presence of antigen and to induce large numbers of Tregs, which can then be transfused back to the patient. The question of antigen specificity here may be less important than previously thought; i.e., it may be possible to expand the Tregs using one or more than one retinal or even nonretinal antigen, since Tregs once induced act in a nonantigen-specific manner. In addition, the notion of bystander tolerance described above suggests that Tregs to one antigen may expand to associated antigens if presented in the right context and vicinity. The availability of spontaneous models of uveoretinitis allows these concepts to be tested with direct relevance to the clinical situation of ongoing disease.

BEDSIDE TO BENCH TO BENCH TO BEDSIDE

There is a current trend for "translational medicine," which encompasses the concept of converting results from experimental studies to clinically relevant treatments for actual diseases, i.e., shifting research from the intellectual pursuit of fundamental mechanisms to practically useful research outcomes. In fact, those working in the field of applied experimental medicine will consider that part of their remit has always been to develop translational medicine. Good examples of these approaches are shown in the early translation of results using cyclosporine A, tacrolimus, anti-TNF-α therapy, and the emergence of interferon-α (IFN-α) for the treatment of retinal vasculitis. The history of IFN-α is unusual. IFN-α was the first cytokine to be isolated and has been in clinical use for many years for the treatment of various conditions, including hepatitis C and certain tumors. At one time it was proposed as an antiangiogenic therapy for age-related macular degeneration, but the clinical evidence was not strong. Its role as an immunostimulant and promoter of systemic autoimmunity is well recognized, but in autoimmune uveoretinitis, it was reported to have an inhibitory effect (19). Accordingly, it was trialed in a very large case series of patients with severe STOI due to Behçet's disease with remarkable effect (20). A second large series confirmed these initial results and since then further reports of its effectiveness in non-Behçet's disease have been reported (21). These clinical results have generated a series of bench investigations to determine how IFN-α has this clinical effect. IFN-α is known to modulate the function of other groups of circulating T cells in several conditions and has similar effects in T cells from patients with uveitis (5).

In this regard, the work on DC in uveitis has opened a reverberating loop of bench to bedside research. IFN-α is known to be produced by many cells in response to viral infection but constitutively only by a rare subset of DC, known as plasmacytoid DC (pDC). It followed therefore that if IFN-α is effective in certain forms of severe uveitis, it may be acting as a replacement therapy and thus perhaps there is an intrinsic defect in IFN-α production by pDC, particularly in pDC from patients with uveitis. This turned out to be the case: patients with uveitis have a reduced number of pDC, which collectively have a significantly reduced ability to secrete IFN-α in response to stimulation by toll receptor ligation (TLR9) (5). Thus, the clinical problem and the experience is leading back toward a more complete understanding of the pathogenesis of the disease which may in turn lead to a better understanding to the role of Tregs under the control of DC and eventually better treatments.

CONCLUSION

This Chapter has described a few of the many research questions which are raised by the clinical problem of sight-threatening uveitis and ocular inflammation. We hope it also highlights the importance of such research questions in helping us understand the basis of immune tolerance and how it breaks down in autoimmune disease. The value of animal models discussed and the particular value and insights which can be gained from the ocular models for immunological studies has in the past led to the current immunotherapies which we use and will in the future deliver hopefully more promising therapies.

REFERENCES

1. Jabs DA, Nussenblatt RB, Rosenbaum JT. Standardization of uveitis nomenclature for reporting clinical data. Results of the First International Workshop. Am J Ophthalmol 2005; 140(3):509–516.

2. Kilmartin DJ, Fletcher ZJ, Almeida JA, et al. CD69 expression on peripheral CD4+ T cells parallels disease activity and is reduced by mycophenolate mofetil therapy in uveitis. Invest Ophthalmol Vis Sci 2001; 42(6):1285–1292.

3. Curnow SJ, Falciani F, Durrani OM, et al. Multiplex bead immunoassay analysis of aqueous humor reveals distinct cytokine profiles in uveitis. Invest Ophthalmol Vis Sci 2005; 46(11):4251–4259.

4. Murphy CC, Duncan L, Forrester JV, et al. Systemic CD4(+) T cell phenotype and activation status in intermediate uveitis. Br J Ophthalmol 2004; 88(3):412–426.

5. Plskova J, Greiner K, Muckersie E, et al. Interferon-alpha: a key factor in autoimmune disease? Invest Ophthalmol Vis Sci 2006; 47(9):3946–3950.

6. Nussenblatt RB, Palestine AG, Rook AH, et al. Treatment of intraocular inflammatory disease with cyclosporin A. Lancet 1983; 2(8344):235–238.

7. Stockinger B, Veldhoen M. Differentiation and function of Th17 T cells. Curr Opin Immunol 2007; 19(3):281–286 (review).

8. Wacker WB, Lipton MM. Experimental allergic uveitis: homologous retina as uveitogenic antigen. Nature 1965; 206 (981):253–254.

9. Forrester JV, Liversidge J, Dua HS, et al. Comparison of clinical and experimental uveitis. Curr Eye Res 1990; 9(suppl):75–84 (review).

10. Gocho K, Kondo I, Yamaki K. Identification of autoreactive T cells in Vogt-Koyanagi-Harada disease. Invest Ophthalmol Vis Sci 2001; 42(9):2004–2009.

11. Lambe T, Leung JC, Ferry H, et al. Limited peripheral T cell anergy predisposes to retinal autoimmunity. J Immunol 2007; 178(7):4276–4283.

12. Lim WK, Chee SP, Sng I, et al. Immunopathology of progressive subretinal fibrosis: a variant of sympathetic ophthalmia. Am J Ophthalmol 2004; 138(3):475–477.

13. DeVoss J, Hou Y, Johannes K, et al. Spontaneous autoimmunity prevented by thymic expression of a single self-antigen. J Exp Med 2006; 203(12):2727–2735.

14. Broderick CA, Smith AJ, Balaggan KS, et al. Local administration of an adeno-associated viral vector expressing IL-10 reduces monocyte infiltration and subsequent photoreceptor damage during experimental autoimmune uveitis. Mol Ther 2005; 12(2):369–373.

15. Bloquel C, Bejjani R, Bigey P, et al. Plasmid electrotransfer of eye ciliary muscle: principles and therapeutic efficacy using hTNF-alpha soluble receptor in uveitis. FASEB J 2006; 20(2):389–391.

16. Gocke AR, Cravens PD, Ben LH, et al. T-bet regulates the fate of Th1 and Th17 lymphocytes in autoimmunity. J Immunol 2007; 178(3):1341–1348.

17. Jiang HR, Muckersie E, Robertson M, et al. Antigen-specific inhibition of experimental autoimmune uveoretinitis by bone marrow-derived immature dendritic cells. Invest Ophthalmol Vis Sci 2003; 44(4):1598–1607.

18. Siepmann K, Biester S, Plsková J, et al. CD4+CD25+ T regulatory cells induced by LPS-activated bone marrow dendritic cells suppress experimental autoimmune uveoretinitis in vivo. Graefes Arch Clin Exp Ophthalmol 2007; 245(2):221–229.

19. Mizuguchi J, Takeuchi M, Usui M. Type I interferons as immunoregulatory molecules; implications for therapy in experimental autoimmune uveoretinitis. Arch Immunol Ther Exp (Warsz) 2002; 50(4):243–254.

20. Kotter I, Eckstein AK, Stübiger N, et al. Treatment of ocular symptoms of Behçet's disease with interferon alpha 2a: a pilot study. Br J Ophthalmol 1998; 82(5):488–494.

21. Plskova J, Greiner K, Forrester JV. Interferon-alpha as an effective treatment for noninfectious posterior uveitis and panuveitis. Am J Ophthalmol 2007; 144(1): 55–61.

22. Bizheva K, Pflug R, Hermann B, et al. Optophysiology: depth-resolved probing of retinal physiology with functional ultrahigh-resolution optical coherence tomography. Proc Natl Acad Sci U S A 2006; 103(13):5066–5071.

Index

Milton Keynes UK
Ingram Content Group UK Ltd.
UKHW050451071024
449327UK00015B/334